Zen Martinoli's

5 Minute
Fitness

Maximum benefit – minimum effort

First published in paperback in...

JOHN BLAKE

Published by Metro Publishing
an imprint of John Blake Publishing Ltd
3 Bramber Court, 2 Bramber Road,
London W14 9PB, England

www.johnblakepublishing.co.uk

www.facebook.com/Johnblakepub facebook
twitter.com/johnblakepub twitter

... paperback ... in 2011

ISBN 978 1 84358 383 7

British Library Cataloguing-in-Publication Data

A catalogue record for this book is available from the British Library.

Design by www.envydesign.co.uk

Printed in Great Britain by CPI Bookmarque, Croydon CR0 4TD

1 3 5 7 9 10 8 6 4 2

© Text copyright Zen Martinoli
Exercise photographs © Michele Martinoli
www.michelemartinoli.com

Papers used by John Blake Publishing are natural, recyclable products made from
wood grown in sustainable forests. The manufacturing processes conform to the
environmental regulations of the country of origin.

Acknowledgements

I would like to thank my mother, Michele, for her contribution to *5 Minute Fitness* – your hard work and dedication to this project have been greatly appreciated, both in shooting the exercises but also the huge amount of time it took you to edit all the images!

Thank you to Lisa, Richard and Edward for your valuable time and perfectly executed exercise instruction visuals! You were all very patient and brilliantly professional models.

Gratitude to all of those who believed in the concept of *5 Minute Fitness*, supported, encouraged and made it happen.

Contents

Safety advice
It is important that you consult your doctor before attempting any of the workouts in this book if you are just starting out on physical activity. If you have any underlying medical health issues or biomechanical deficiencies (problems with joints), a heart condition or high blood pressure it is essential that you get the relevant clearance. Use the workouts sensibly and should you feel pain at any point, stop exercising. It is important to make a clear distinction between feeling the discomfort of intense exercise and exacerbating a problem by continuing. Avoid exercise when suffering any temporary ailments, such as colds, fevers, etc.

Chapter One

INTRODUCTION TO THE MINI-WORKOUT

Important: Due to the nature of mini-workouts being high in intensity (level of difficulty), they are not suitable for the complete beginner, unfit or sedentary person. If you fall into this category, please read the introduction to physical fitness (Chapter Two) before attempting any of the subsequent levels, which will give you a rounded idea as to why and how the mini-workouts are approached. Within this chapter the individual components of fitness are explored in detail as well as the benefits derived from them in isolation. This book, however, incorporates all of these aspects of fitness targeted simultaneously.

What is the Mini-Workout?

Within these pages is a wide variety of short, high-intensity workouts which can be employed anywhere, at any time and with no equipment required except for a timer/stopwatch in some instances. All workouts use only bodyweight and are suitable for both men and women who are free of injury or biomechanical limitations and have no underlying medical issues.

This book is not intended to replace your current exercise programme (if you have one!) but will instead enhance and complement it. Used correctly, however, it could in itself provide a perfectly sufficient workload to maintain and gain health and fitness benefits. Its intended use is for people who find it hard to get to the gym or for those away on trips who want to sustain their current fitness levels conveniently in their own time and with no equipment.

The mini-workouts are designed to accommodate occasional exercisers through to advanced exercisers. There are three levels in total with progressions throughout each level. Although these workouts are not sports-specific, the intention is to hit all areas of fitness within the limitations of time and equipment, improving anaerobic and aerobic fitness while building lean muscle and burning fat.

The terms aerobic and anaerobic refer to energy pathways that are utilised during exercise. Different types of activity will determine which energy systems are engaged to produce energy for the working muscles. In order to improve aerobic or anaerobic fitness, one must engage in the specific types of activities associated with each as explained here:

Aerobic means 'with oxygen'
This energy system is activated during prolonged periods of activity in order to sustain continuous exercise, often referred to as 'steady state' or 'continuous'. During aerobic exercise, the body creates energy by utilising oxygen in a complex and gradual chemical process to break down glucose which in turn releases energy. Long-distance running, jogging and cycling are typical examples of aerobic exercise.

Anaerobic means 'without oxygen'
The anaerobic system is activated during short, explosive bouts of activity. This instant demand requires a more rapid chemical process to take place whereby energy is derived from the short supply of stored body chemicals without the use of oxygen. Sprinting and weightlifting are typical examples of anaerobic exercises.

Fitness propagates fitness and so the more you acquire, the quicker the gains. Being able to work at a consistently higher level is the key to unlocking the door to your true physical potential.

The *5 Minute Fitness* workouts have been designed to exploit minimum time into maximum benefit with minimum effort. Don't be misled by 'minimum effort' as this relates to the volume of time spent working out: you will be required to put considerable effort into the allotted time frame per workout.

So, how can short workouts be effective? It has been widely accepted for many years that in order to burn calories/fat you have to train aerobically for an extended period of time (twenty minutes or more) at a moderate intensity as, during this time, fat is metabolised as fuel. However, research now shows high-intensity exercise produces up to nine times more fat-loss benefit for every calorie burned than low-intensity exercise.

Why is high-intensity training more effective at burning fat than long, moderate aerobic training? It's all to do with a four-letter acronym: EPOC (Excess Post-Exercise Oxygen Consumption), a scientific way of describing the calories you burn post-exercise.

During aerobic exercise you only burn calories while you work, utilising fat as fuel over an extended period at a moderate to low intensity. However, with high-intensity exercise (even as short as four minutes at a time), your body continues to burn calories for up to two days more, repaying the oxygen debt to your muscles and making this method much more efficient in terms of time investment versus calories burned.

These workouts are designed so that you can dip in and out as you please but are not intended as a programme. Instead, they should be used to supplement those times when you are away on trips or during periods when you can't make the gym. If you prefer to use the book as a stand-alone guide, I will make recommendations as to frequency of use and which workouts should be employed (and when) at the beginning of each level. The primary intention of this book is to encourage maximum benefits to fitness in minimal time and the protocols below are a feature of each level. All can be considered as being under the umbrella of high-intensity training, so let's take a closer look.

GPP (General Physical Preparedness) or General Fitness Training

GPP training originates from the Russian system of coaching athletes designed to target those areas of fitness neglected when training sports-specifically for an event. It was discovered by increasing an athlete's GPP enhanced overall performance – for example, in the case of a power-lifter, GPP training would consist of anything other than power-lifting or maximal strength work. In essence, GPP means 'all-round fitness', the intention being to create a broad base of fitness for the athlete or exerciser. It's important to note that if you do train sports specifically, it is good practice to adopt this approach as it encourages balance and strength in all areas.

GPP is particularly useful in terms of the mini-workout as this is precisely what this book sets out to achieve: maintenance and development of all-round fitness. I have used this protocol in both timed and repetition form; some of the featured workouts will be in timed intervals, while others are in sets of predetermined repetitions. These are challenging, intense and engaging workouts and the level of difficulty increases as you work through the levels.

The Benefits of GPP
- Improves aerobic conditioning and VO2 Max *
- Anaerobic conditioning is improved
- Improves speed and power
- Agility (motor skill) is improved
- Improves body composition
- Co-ordination (motor skill) is improved
- Promotes fat loss.

Bodyweight Circuits
This form of GPP will typically include six to eight different exercises per circuit with some working smaller muscles in isolation, whereas

---

*The maximum amount of oxygen an individual utilises during intense or maximal exercise (VO2 Max) is expressed in terms of millilitres of oxygen consumed per kilogram of body weight per minute. It is commonly used to determine aerobic (cardiovascular) fitness. Aerobic fitness relates to how well your heart, lungs and organs work when transporting and utilising oxygen in your body. As aerobic fitness levels increase, so too does VO2 Max and with it, the body's ability to efficiently deliver and distribute oxygen to the working muscles and this results in improved performance levels.

The most accurate way to measure your VO2 Max is to perform a maximal exercise stress test in a laboratory. There are, however, other more simple ways of calculating your VO2 Max without resorting to using complicated apparatus in a science laboratory. If you are still intrigued, I've included a link to a simplified online VO2 Max calculator: www.shapesense.com/fitness-exercise/calculators/vo2max-calculator.aspx. Further investigation on the Internet will provide you with a variety of other methods.

standard GPP workouts typically include four compound exercises (multi-joint movements). Both are extremely effective in developing all-round fitness. Bodyweight circuits also incorporate a combination of muscular strength and endurance including Plyometrics (used to develop speed, strength/power) and Isometrics (a form of strength training) plus core exercises. These are challenging and intense.

The Benefits of Bodyweight Circuits
- Improves aerobic conditioning
- Anaerobic conditioning is improved
- Improves speed and power
- Agility (motor skill) is improved
- Improves body composition
- Co-ordination is improved
- Promotes fat loss.

HIIT (High-Intensity Interval Training) Using Tabata Protocol
HIIT workouts typically consist of work intervals of high-intensity exercise followed by intervals of medium- or low-intensity exercise. This form of training is taxing yet yields great benefits in terms of fitness and fat loss.

What is Tabata?
Tabata training is the single most effective type of high-intensity interval training. The Tabata Workout was invented by Dr Izumi Tabata and his team at the National Institute of Fitness and Sports in Tokyo: their research centred on establishing a protocol which would optimally target anaerobic and aerobic conditioning. After much experimentation they discovered that the following protocol was the most effective:

- Work: Twenty seconds (100 per cent maximum effort)
- Rest: Ten seconds
- Eight cycles
- Total: Four minutes.

Studies showed improvements of 28 per cent in anaerobic capacity as well as a substantial increase in aerobic capacity, making Tabata great for fat loss, plus anaerobic and aerobic energy systems are both improved. As a training method, this is extremely taxing and must be approached with caution: training all out for a period of twenty seconds is challenge for anyone, let alone repeating the process a further seven times!

Important: A word of advice when approaching intensity with Tabata. A good start would be to adopt 'relative intensity' so begin by doing intervals at say, 80 per cent max and work towards 100 per cent. Rest longer between sets and attempt perhaps two to three sets to begin with. If you have a history of heart disease, have high cholesterol or high blood pressure or have been leading a sedentary lifestyle, please consult your doctor before attempting this type of training. Also, ensure you cool down properly and allow your breathing to return to normal: stopping suddenly after ultra high-intensity (or any high-intensity exercise) may leave you feeling dizzy and cause you to suffer muscle pain. Tabata will be adopted in Levels 2 and 3 (pages 151 and 173) and performed using the large muscle groups.

The Benefits of High-Intensity Training and Tabata Protocol

• Highly effective in improving anaerobic conditioning
• Also highly effective in improving aerobic conditioning
• Extremely short workout times
• Highly effective fat burner
• Improves speed and power
• Co-ordination and agility are improved.

Muscular Strength and Endurance Training

To a certain extent, all the workouts will include elements of muscular strength and endurance. At higher levels, the introduction of Isometrics and Plyometrics will add a further challenge for the more conditioned individual. There are advanced mini-workouts in Levels 2 and 3 focusing specifically on these areas. Chapter Two contains more detail on Plyometrics and Isometrics.

The Benefits of the Mini-Workout

- Cost-effective and time saving, this is a great workout in a fraction of the time you spend in a gym!
- Mini-workouts are easier to plan and can be performed anywhere, at any time so they are extremely convenient.
- Many scientific studies have proved that short, intense workouts are hugely beneficial in metabolising fat and increasing levels of fitness.
- A study in the Journal of Applied Physiology (2007) showed that those who did short workouts with rest periods in between burned more fat than others who carried out longer, more sustained workouts.
- Scientific research shows alternating short intervals of intense activity with brief rest periods delivers more benefit for less exercise. As a way of building fitness and muscle power it surpasses traditional types of long-term exercise such as cycling or walking.
- After even a brief workout, stress levels are reduced: not only are endorphins (mood-elevating hormones) released, but Cortisol (a stress hormone) is also burnt.
- All mini-workouts can be adjusted to the average person
- The mini-workout book enables those who are seriously into their exercise to maintain fitness levels while away on holidays or business trips.
- When you work out intensely, you will achieve bigger gains than if you perform slow, low-intensity workouts dragged out over a period of time. Essentially, with shorter workouts, the return on investment is far greater.
- Muscular strength and endurance are improved, as are motor skills in terms of power, agility, co-ordination and reaction time.
- Body image and self-esteem are enhanced.

Chapter Two

INTRODUCTION TO PHYSICAL FITNESS

If this is your first foray into the world of fitness or you have been leading a practically sedentary lifestyle up until now, it's important to address in detail how to create a safe platform upon which to build. Physical fitness is incremental and without employing too many overused analogies, good preparation, solid foundation and correct construction must be ensured to create a robust structure with all the contents in peak condition!

There are five components to physical fitness – muscular endurance, muscular strength, cardiovascular fitness, flexibility (health related) and motor fitness (skill related) – however it is important to acknowledge that our 'total fitness' is comprised of other elements such as emotional, social, spiritual, mental and nutritional factors, all of which are inextricably linked and instrumental to leading a quality, well-balanced and nourished existence. Our focus for the purpose of this book will centre on the physical aspects.

There are important factors which affect your physical fitness: we have our own blueprint to begin with in terms of body type and genetic make-up, with some people having more of a propensity for their bodies to respond to training than others. Also, what we consume, how active we are, our age and our current state of health have a direct relationship on our physical fitness as a whole. However, we can reverse the effects of aging through exercise, change what we consume, alter our lifestyles and eliminate abusive habits, all leading to a heightened level of physical fitness.

Health-related Fitness
- Cardiovascular fitness
- Muscular strength
- Muscular endurance
- Flexibility
- Motor fitness (skill-related fitness)
- Promotes agility, co-ordination, reaction time, power, speed and balance.

The health-related components have a direct impact on health, body image and general well-being whereas motor fitness covers the ability level in which muscles respond during physical tasks. To best understand the impact exercise has on us physically, it is advantageous to take a closer look at these areas of fitness, bar flexibility, which is covered in the pre- and post-exercise Chapter Three.

The body responds physiologically in precise ways to different types of stimulus: activity, intensity (level of difficulty) and duration of exercise (time). Depending on how we approach them, these variables will yield specific results and are directly related to our fitness levels and/or fitness objectives. Full understanding of the fundamentals will give you greater insight as to how the mini-workouts are approached in each level described in this book. The following pages will cover:
- Energy production
- Energy systems
- Aerobic training
- Anaerobic and core training
- Motor fitness

Energy Production
All the functions of the body require energy and as we begin to exercise, we must produce more energy than at rest. Energy is derived from the food we store in our bodies, the main sources being as follows:

Carbohydrate: Stored as glycogen in our liver and muscles, which is subsequently broken down to glucose and can be used as fuel by all tissues in the body; utilised for short-term energy during high-intensity exercise.

Fat: Stored as adipose tissue under the skin and around the organs. Fat is broken down to fatty acids to release energy; utilised for long-term energy during moderate exercise.

Protein: Often called the 'building blocks', protein is used for the growth and repair of tissues in the body and is not stored in the same way as fat or carbohydrate. It is broken down into amino acids to provide energy, which occurs only in prolonged bouts of activity when glycogen stores are in short supply: for example, in the latter stages of an endurance event.

So how does the body produce energy, what gets used and when? Carbohydrate, fat and to a lesser extent, protein (in emergencies) are broken down by various chemical processes and stored within the muscles to produce the same end product: an energy-rich compound called Adenosine Triphosphate (ATP) – the body's 'energy currency'. ATP is a small molecule comprised of one part Adenosine and three parts Phosphate connected by high-energy phosphate bonds.

The energy locked within the phosphate bonds is released when one of the phosphate groups splits away to become Adenosine Diphosphate (ADP). This energy results predominantly in body heat (we get hotter as we exercise), the remainder being used to service every requirement we have from muscle contraction to digestion.

Once energy has been released, ADP will be re-synthesised back to ATP in a continuous cycle of energy production (the ATP Cycle), similar to a re-chargeable battery expending energy then being 're-charged' by the breakdown of fuel. As we start to exercise, the body's demand for the initial short supply of ATP increases and so the manufacture of ATP is elevated.

The ATP Cycle

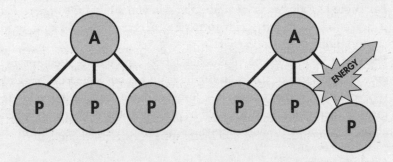

(A) ATP molecule (Adenosine Triphosphate)   (B) ATP breakdown to release energy

The Energy Systems

ATP or energy can be created in three different ways, defined as energy systems. Each has a different pathway and speed in which it produces energy. At any one time our reserves of ATP are minimal, so depending on what the demand is (intensity and duration) will determine which energy system comes into play and under what conditions it is created:

ATP-PC (Phosphocreatine System/without oxygen)

LA (Lactic Acid or Anaerobic System/without oxygen)

Aerobic (with oxygen).

ATP-PC System

The ATP-PC system creates ATP at an exceptionally fast rate to facilitate maximal bursts of energy lasting no more than eight to ten seconds. ATP is created without the use of oxygen and utilises a high-energy compound stored within the muscle cells called phosphocreatine (PC). As PC breaks down to release energy for muscle contraction, ADP is rapidly assimilated back to ATP. However, limited amounts of creatine (which originates from the liver) quickly render the ATP-PC system redundant. Examples of sports when the ATP-PC System is used include: 100 metres sprint, maximal weight lift, long jump and anything of an explosive nature.

Lactic Acid System

After PC stores are depleted, the predominant system becomes the Lactic Acid or Anaerobic Glycolytic system, enabling you to continue to exercise at a very high intensity for up to ninety seconds. The process itself utilises glycogen (stored within the muscles) broken down to glucose to produce ATP in the absence of oxygen; the result of this rapid conversion minus oxygen is the by-product lactic acid. The onset of lactic acid causes fatigue and muscle soreness and eventually results in being forced to drop the intensity or stop altogether. Examples of sports when used include: 400 to 800 metre sprint or weight training 'set'.

Aerobic System

After a few minutes the body switches from anaerobic to aerobic. The aerobic system creates ATP in the presence of oxygen from the breakdown of both carbohydrate (glycogen) and fat (fatty acids) at a slower rate than its predecessor anaerobic systems. Demand for energy is gradual during aerobic activity as the body can engage in this more complex (but more efficient) process and produce up to twenty times more energy than before. The use of fatty acids becomes the dominant fuel as aerobic exercise is performed at a lower intensity for a prolonged period: the higher the intensity becomes, the more glycogen is used. Examples of sports when used include long distance events and any prolonged and sustained activity.

Energy systems and fuels used at the time of exertion

Exercise Time	Main Energy	Intensity	Fuel Used
1–10 seconds	ATP-PC	Maximal	ATP and Phosphocreatine
Up to 30 seconds	ATP-PC and lactic acid	Very high	ATP-PC and Glycogen
Up to 90 seconds	Lactic acid	Very high	Glycogen
1.30–3.00 minutes	Lactic acid and aerobic	High	Glycogen
3.00+ minutes	Aerobic	Moderate to high	Glycogen and Adipose tissue (fatty acids)

The consumption of Adipose tissue (fat) as fuel becomes predominant in aerobic exercise when the intensity is moderate and prolonged in duration. This is the traditional approach to burning calories/fat, though not the most effective on a time-versus-results basis*, however it is a less strenuous and more appropriate approach for the unconditioned individual.

So far we have outlined the energy systems in isolation but in reality, all three are used during exercise. The type of activity, intensity and duration will determine which energy system the emphasis is placed on. Certain sports, for example, are predominantly anaerobic (sprints, throwing, jumping) whereas others are predominantly aerobic (distance running, cycling, swimming). Most sports are a combination of all three to a greater or lesser degree.

In boxing, for example, aerobic is the main system used (so long as the fight lasts a few rounds!) as the boxer will sustain continuous, rhythmical movements throughout interspersed with intermittent explosive punches and combinations, sporadically engaging both ATP-PC and lactic systems. A boxer is a perfect example of an athlete who has high levels of cross-fitness similarly to a footballer or rugby player (depending on the position played).

The majority of sports require a level of cross-fitness as all energy systems are used, however for extremely specific sports such as a 100m sprint, an athlete's ability to perform long distances would not be required; training focus would be placed on maximal speed, strength and power.

The mini-workouts within this book encompass all energy systems, however emphasis will be placed (especially in Levels 2 and 3) on high-intensity intervals and circuits. As explained earlier, the aim is to create short workouts with maximum benefit in minimal time and to this effect they are required by nature to be very challenging. A five-minute stroll for the unfit or sedentary person may provide a useful platform from which to start but for the more conditioned exerciser would be of little benefit and would represent a 'light' warm-up.

---

*Reference EPOC (Excess Post-exercise Oxygen Consumption) for benefits of High-Intensity Interval Training (see Introduction to the Mini-Workout, Chapter One).

Let's take a look at the types of exercise associated with aerobic and anaerobic fitness.

Aerobic (Cardiovascular) Fitness

Definition: The ability of your heart, lungs and organs to consume, transport and utilise oxygen. As we become fitter, our bodies become more efficient at this process. This is commonly measured as your VO2 Max or Maximal Oxygen Uptake.

Cardiovascular exercise is any physical activity using the large muscles of the body in rhythmic, continuous motion. The benefits of aerobic training include the following:

• Increases organ function
• Strengthens and improves efficiency of heart and lungs
• Increases bone density
• Reduces risk of diabetes and heart disease
• Burns calories/fat and raises your metabolic rate
• Increases muscle endurance
• Also increases capillary density, enabling more blood to flow
  to the muscles
• Relieves anxiety, depression and stress
• Release mood-elevating hormones (endorphins)
• Sleeping patterns and self-image are improved

To get started, we need to establish an appropriate training zone that will improve our cardiovascular fitness. The principle is to create an overload on the system which is a little out of our comfort zone: as our fitness improves, the parameters of that comfort zone change and we are able to work at a higher rate and increase the intensity (level of difficulty) and frequency of our workouts.

Use Your Heart Rate to find Your Aerobic Training Zones

In the case of aerobic exercise, the level of intensity can be measured using your heart rate. With the use of a heart-rate monitor, you will be able to keep track of your heart rate and stay within the zone most suited to your level of fitness and goals. An alternative method for measuring intensity called RPE (Rate of Perceived Exertion) is explained further on (page 18). Study both methods for a full understanding of the training zones and their benefits and how they relate to each other.

In order to establish training zones using heart rate, it is necessary to determine MHR (Maximum Heart Rate), which measures how fast your heart can beat or contract in one minute. Various formulae are available and some more accurate than others. For the purposes of the exercises in this book, we will use the most common and simple age-adjusted formula (although not entirely accurate, plus or minus 12 beats either side and typically slightly less accurate for women). If you want to find a more precise formula, many are available on the Internet, for example: http://nowlin.com/heartrate.htm
http://www.brianmac.co.uk/maxhr.htm

The age-adjusted MHR for a 40-year-old would be 180 MHR: (220 – your age = x). For example, 220 – 40 = 180 beats per minute (BPM).

With our approximate MHR we can now become acquainted with the different heart zones, which are measured in percentages of your MHR. Aerobic training zones are considered to be between 50 and 80 per cent of your MHR, after which we move into anaerobic training. Here are some examples calculated on an MHR of 180:

50 per cent of 180 = 90 BPM
60 per cent of 180 = 108 BPM
70 per cent of 180 = 126 BPM
80 per cent of 180 = 144 BPM
90 per cent of 180 = 162 BPM.

In the case of MHR being 180 and as a beginner, you would be working in Zone 1 (keeping your heart rate between 50 and 60 per cent of MHR, translating to 90 to108 BPM). The exercise zones are detailed below: the body becomes more efficient and capable of increasing intensity of exercise as it adapts to overload.

Fox and Haskell Formula

		20	25	30	35	40	45	50	55	65	70
	100%	200	195	190	185	180	175	170	165	155	150
	90%	180	176	171	167	162	158	153	149	140	135
	80%	160	156	152	148	144	140	136	132	124	120
	70%	140	137	133	130	126	123	119	116	109	105
	60%	120	117	114	111	108	105	102	99	93	90
	50%	100	98	95	93	90	88	85	83	78	75

EXERCISE ZONES / AGE — BEATS PER MINUTE

Zones: VO2 Max (Maximum effort); Anaerobic (Hardcore training); Aerobic (Cardio training / Endurance); Weight control (Fitness / Fat burn); Moderate activity (Maintenance / Warm up)

50 to 60 Per Cent MHR (Moderate Activity Zone)

This zone is often used as a warm-up phase for more conditioned athletes. It represents a comfortable level of intensity for the beginner or unfit person to start at and increase fitness levels and so begin to burn fat.

60 to 70 Per Cent MHR (Weight Control or Weight Management Zone)

In this zone, stored body fat becomes the primary source of energy; hence weight control. An ideal zone for slow, long-distance exercise working at a moderate level of intensity suitable for the majority of people: the heart's ability to pump blood begins to benefit more here as does the muscles' ability to utilise oxygen.

70 to 80 Per Cent MHR (Fitness and Endurance Zone)

This is the most effective zone for improving cardiovascular fitness and generally referred to as the 'Aerobic Zone' or 'Target Zone'. It represents the optimal zone to increase cardio-respiratory capacity (the ability to transport oxygenated blood to the muscle cells). As you become fitter, you will be able to cover more distance in less time.

80 to 90 Per Cent MHR (Aerobic into Anaerobic Zone)

Once you reach approximately 85 per cent MHR, you move from one source of energy production to another, referred to as the Anaerobic Threshold (AT*). This is the point at which the body cannot effectively remove lactic acid from the working muscles quickly enough as the AT is elevated through adaptation and the body's ability to metabolise lactic acid is increased. This zone would be characterised as hard, resulting in tired muscles, heavy breathing and fatigue.

90 to 100 per cent MHR (Anaerobic/Maximum Effort/VO2 Max Zone)

This zone should be attempted only by very fit individuals: lactic acid is quickly produced with an oxygen debt to the muscles. Periods of exercise are short in duration and suited to explosive bursts.

Rating of Perceived Exertion (RPE)

> **Important:** When using RPE, it is important that you distinguish between the effects of physical fatigue and danger signs such as shortness of breath or dizziness. Always monitor yourself properly and if in doubt, stop.

There is an alternative way to calculate intensity without equipment but this relies on an accurate personal appraisal of how hard you are pushing yourself. RPE (Rating of Perceived Exertion) is a scale whereby the intensity you are working at is perceived in terms of numbers 0–10*

---

*Anaerobic Threshold (AT) is the point at which lactic acid (a waste product produced by the anaerobic system) begins to accumulate in the bloodstream during exercise inhibiting performance. More conditioned exercisers have a higher AT, which enables them to train at a higher intensity for longer periods because their bodies have become accustomed to removing lactic acid at a rate fast enough to continue exercising whereas the unconditioned person's body will be less efficient and reach their AT far sooner. More information provided in Chapter Two.

*G. Borg, 'Perceived Exertion as an Indicator of Somatic Stress', Scandinavian Journal of Rehabilitation Medicine 1970, 2(2), 92–98.

The original scale was 6–20, however a simpler version of 0–10 is widely adopted and also known as Borg CR10 Scale.

Although not entirely scientific, if you are honest with your own feedback then RPE can be an effective indicator of intensity and may be broken down into 'zones'. According to research, numbers 3–7 correlate approximately to 50 to 90 per cent on the MHR chart.

Borg CR10 Scale

0	Nothing at all
0.5	Extremely weak (just noticeable)
1	Very weak
2	Weak (light)
3	Moderate
4	Somewhat strong
5	Strong (heavy)
6	
7	Very strong
8	
9	
10	Extremely strong
*	Maximal

Some more feedback on how you feel and how this relates to the scale:

3 Moderate: Easy to perform

4 Somewhat strong: Fairly easy

5 Strong (heavy): Breathing and working a little hard

6 Stronger: Beginning to breathe heavily

7 Very strong: Very challenging, breathing very hard

8 Working and breathing seriously hard

9 Approaching upper limits, working and breathing at near maximal intensity

10 Extremely strong: Working and breathing at maximal intensity

Frequency and Duration of Workouts

For the unconditioned or unfit person, it is recommended that you perform short sessions of about fifteen to twenty minutes of moderate intensity and build up frequency and session length as your fitness improves. The 'frequency' is how many times you exercise in a week, 'intensity' is how hard you are going to train and the 'length' will be for how long. So a good place to begin would be: Frequency: three times week, Intensity: 50 to 60 per cent MHR, Length: fifteen to twenty minutes. As your fitness improves, you can then progress by upping each of these categories.

CV Training

There are various methods of CV training and we will cover them in detail. The first is Steady State/Continuous Training/Interval Training and for the purposes of this book, we will deal with what can be achieved with bodyweight alone. If you attend a gym, machines such as treadmills, rowing machines, bicycles, etc. will have pre-programmed workouts which include Continuous or Steady State, Interval and Fartlek training (Fartlek training comes from the Swedish for 'Speed Play' and essentially is training over any distance at randomised speeds, combining both aerobic and anaerobic systems). Also, you can switch between different types of equipment to mix up your sessions to produce a cross-training experience but here, we will focus simply on bodyweight and a 'low-tech' approach.

Steady State or Continuous Training

This involves you training for a set period of time while maintaining a steady pace (or constant intensity) and remaining in your training zone. It can be as simple as going for ten-minute walk and maintaining a steady pace to suit you. This type of training presents the perfect starting point for beginners to build a platform of fitness and easily measure improvement. As your fitness improves, you will be able to exercise for longer and/or increase intensity.

Continuous Training is categorised as Continuous Short (up to one hour) or Continuous Long (one hour plus – normally used as a sports-specific conditioner, i.e. for long-distance runners). Here is an example:
• Warm-up three to five minutes (gradual build-up in intensity)

- Ten minutes of moderate intensity (walking at Level 3–4 using RPE)
- Cool down for three to five minutes (gradual cool in intensity).

Interval Training

Interval workouts involve alternating higher-intensity or moderate exercise (work sets) with low-intensity recovery periods (active recovery sets), intensity and recovery being relative to the fitness levels and goals of the individual.

There are different types of Interval training: Aerobic Intervals and High Intensity Intervals (HIIT) – (High Intensity Interval Training/Anaerobic) – predominantly used sports specifically by well-conditioned exercisers or athletes. Levels 2 and 3 (pages 151 and 173) will incorporate various forms of HIIT training.

Please note the difference between alternating higher-intensity exercise with low-intensity recovery periods as opposed to actual high intensity, which in HIIT training is intended as 'ultra' high and using the RPE scale would inhabit Levels 8–*Maximal, not suitable for unconditioned people.

Although both types of Interval training are suited to the regular and/or experienced exerciser, in theory there is no reason why intervals cannot be used by the beginner, unfit or sedentary person: this would simply mean your personal 'Higher Interval' would be higher than your low-intensity recovery period, giving you an Interval training experience.

Aerobic Intervals are characterised as having longer moderate/higher-intensity 'work sets' and longer recovery periods, whereas HIIT Intervals have far shorter, more intense work sets with shorter recovery periods, in some cases ultra-high intensity as with Tabata Intervals, which require the exerciser to work at maximum capacity for twenty-second sets followed by a short recovery of ten seconds, completing eight sets in total. The Tabata protocol (see also page 5) is used throughout this book and is not to be attempted by the unfit or unconditioned exerciser until a sufficient level of fitness has been attained.

Example of a Standard Aerobic Interval

These intervals could constitute jogging for three minutes at moderate/high intensity and walking for three minutes' recovery (low intensity) for those new to exercise. Alternatively for the more conditioned individual, the work interval may be running at a high intensity and jogging in recovery for three minutes:

- Three- to five-minute warm-up
- Three minutes moderate/higher intensity, then three minutes low intensity
- Repeat three to eight times
- Three- to five-minute cool down.

Example of a Standard Aerobic Interval Using RPE Based on Three Intervals

- Three- to five-minute warm-up (gradual build-up to target intensity)
- Three minutes moderate/higher intensity (4–5 RPE) followed by three minutes low intensity (3–4 RPE)
- Three minutes moderate/higher intensity (4–5 RPE) followed by three minutes low intensity (3–4 RPE)
- Three minutes moderate/higher intensity (4–5 RPE) followed by three minutes low intensity (3–4 RPE)
- Three- to five-minute cool down (gradual reduction in intensity).

As you can see, this type of interval approach could be adopted by those new to exercise working within comfortable parameters of intensity as above or by the conditioned athlete (distance runner, for example) working at a higher level of intensity for longer intervals. Below are some examples of High Intensity Interval sessions (Aerobic/Anaerobic). The amount of intervals is for illustrative purposes as a full session may consist of as many as twenty intervals:

- Five-minute warm-up
- Thirty seconds high intensity followed by thirty seconds low intensity
- Thirty seconds high intensity followed by thirty seconds low intensity
- Thirty seconds high intensity followed by thirty seconds low intensity
- Thirty seconds high intensity followed by thirty seconds low intensity
- Five-minute cool down.

Typically, High-Intensity Intervals would constitute activities such as sprinting followed by an active recovery period of walking or jogging. HIIT can also be performed with exercises such as Burpees, Jumping Jacks, Squat Thrusts, Mountain Climbers and Squats among others and these will be extensively employed as you enter Levels 2–3. (See Index of Exercises, Chapter Three)

This approach to Interval Training is geared towards sports conditioning or the experienced exerciser who seeks maximum benefits in a shorter time frame. There are other forms of Interval Training less linear in design, yet still with predetermined interval lengths. For example, high-intensity Pyramid Intervals may look like this:

- Five-minute warm-up
- Thirty seconds high intensity followed by thirty seconds low intensity
- Forty seconds high intensity followed by forty seconds low intensity
- Fifty seconds high intensity followed by fifty seconds low intensity
- Sixty seconds high intensity followed by sixty seconds low intensity
- Fifty seconds high intensity followed by fifty seconds low intensity
- Forty seconds high intensity followed by forty seconds low intensity
- Thirty seconds high intensity followed by thirty seconds low intensity
- Five-minute cool down.

The same approach can be adopted for Aerobic Intervals using longer work and recovery sets performed at a lower intensity. In essence, all exercise works within the interval framework. An interval constitutes a 'work' period and this could equally be ten press-ups followed by a rest period (maybe twenty seconds): if adhered to properly, ten sets of ten press-ups with twenty-second rest periods would be 'press-up intervals'.

Muscular Strength: ATP-PC System/Muscular Endurance: ATP-PC and Lactic Acid

Definition (Anaerobic): Exercise in which oxygen is used up more quickly than the body is able to replenish inside the working muscle. As a result, muscle fibres have to derive their contractile energy from stored substrates glycogen and phosphocreatine. Resistance training and high-intensity training constitute this form of exercise.

If you are a beginner, unfit or sedentary person, you will make considerable gains with the use of bodyweight as a resistance. For the more experienced exerciser whose main goal is building strength, bodyweight may serve as maintenance or be supplemental to their regular gym workouts.

The Benefits of Muscular Strength and Endurance Training

- Increases physical performance (posture, balance, etc.)
- Decreases blood pressure
- Strengthens bones, so reducing the onset of osteoporosis
- Increases tendon and ligament strength
- Improves overall appearance and body composition
- Increases metabolic efficiency (the ability to burn excess calories)
- Decreased risk of sustaining injury (improved shock-absorbing musculature)
- Reverses muscle wastage - atrophy - which occurs naturally as we age

Let's first define muscular strength and endurance: the logical way to explain the strength continuum is in terms of using resistance equipment. We will then look at how this translates to using bodyweight. Muscle strength may be described as: 'the force that a muscle or muscle group can exert against a resistance in one maximal effort'. Effectively, One Maximum Repetition (1RM) is the heaviest weight a muscle or muscles can overcome in one contraction. Once this figure is established to improve strength, you would use a resistance (nearly maximal) in terms of RM between 1–12RM. So, a 6RM would mean six reps of a resistance you can overcome before muscular failure.

Based on a 1RM of 100kg, your 8RM would be 80kg (80 per cent of 100kg).

Example: Heavy resistance x low repetition = muscular strength
80kg x eight reps = muscular strength.

Muscular endurance may be described as 'the ability of a muscle (or group of muscles) to sustain repeated contractions against a resistance for an extended period'. It is the ability of a muscle (or muscles) to repeatedly contract against a 'sub-maximal' resistance for extended repetitions. This would represent working between 15–25RM.

Based on a 1RM of 100kg, your 20RM would be 20kg (20 per cent of 100kg)

Example: Low resistance x high repetition = muscular endurance
20kg x 20 reps = muscular endurance

As we won't be using resistance equipment, let's look at how muscular strength and endurance relates to using bodyweight only. Using bodyweight presents a more complex challenge and differs from one individual to the next. If an individual can perform ten Standard Press Ups (page 56) then they would be working towards strength gains. On the other hand, if they could perform twenty-five Standard Press Ups then they would find themselves at the other end of the scale in muscular endurance. As resistance cannot be altered with equipment, adjust the level of difficulty with any given exercise by adjusting your body position/angle and modifying the cadence (speed) at which it is performed.

Below is an example of press-up progressions, from easy to the more challenging. The unfit or sedentary individual should begin with a Wall Press Up and if that variation doesn't present much of challenge, graduate up to the Kneeling Press Up, and so on (see also Index of Exercises, pages 45– 132).

Easy to Difficult
Wall Press Up
Kneeling Press Up
Extended Kneeling Press Up
Splayed Leg Press Up
Standard Press Up
One-handed Press Up

If your RM is twenty-five reps using the Kneeling Press Up variation, you will currently be working towards endurance. To increase strength, you must increase the difficulty to a more challenging type of press up. You will soon discover this is an entirely different proposition (remember, you cannot change the resistance as you are working with your own bodyweight) and will only be able to perform minimal reps, landing yourself squarely in the strength zone.

Example: Muscular Endurance Workout Using Bodyweight for the Beginner

Those new to exercising should start from the endurance end of the strength continuum in order to accustom the muscles to resistance and, over time, progress to strength. Muscular endurance may be the 'zone' they wish to remain in, though.

Three- to five-minute warm-up

Exercise	Reps	Sets	Rest between sets in seconds	Rate/Tempo
Kneeling/Wall Press Ups	15–20	2	30–45	Medium
Squats	15–20	2	30–45	Medium
Floor Dips	15–20	2	30–45	Medium
Calf Raises	20–25	2	30–45	Medium
Abdominal Crunches	15–20	2	30–45	Medium
Seated Russian Twist	20	2	30–45	Medium
Dorsal Raises	12–15	2	30–45	Medium

Finally, cool down and stretch.

For instructions on all exercises listed, refer to Index of Exercises in Chapter Four

For instructions on cooling down and stretching, refer to Chapter Three

Workout Notes

Begin by performing Kneeling or Wall Press Ups for one set of fifteen to twenty repetitions. Take a thirty- to forty-five second rest before completing a second set, then rest again and complete Squats, Floor

Dips, Calf Raises, Abdominal Crunches, Russian Twists and Dorsal Raises adopting the same approach for two sets of prescribed repetitions. A medium tempo is smooth and controlled.

To increase the level of difficulty, up the reps/sets, reduce the rest time or modify the exercise to a more challenging variation.

Modification of exercises can also place emphasis on different muscle groups: for example, in the press-up variations below.

Important: Do not attempt any of these until you have established some initial base-strength gains.

- Diamond Press Up: First targets the triceps and then the chest
- Dolphin Press Up: Targets the back, shoulders, arms and core
- Plyometric Press Up: Develops speed strength (power)
- Decline Press Up: Targets upper chest.

(For instructions on all exercises listed, refer to the Index of Exercises in Chapter Four)

The rate (tempo/speed) at which an individual executes an exercise will yield different results. A slower rate engenders strength and growth whereas faster, more explosive movements cultivate speed and strength (power) referred to as 'Plyometrics'. You can also build strength with 'Isometric' contraction of the muscle involving no movement (see below for these techniques). Both are employed throughout this book.

Plyometrics

This type of training originates from Russia and was developed so that athletes could produce fast and powerful movements. The technique involves muscles being loaded, then contracted in rapid sequence: the outcome is being able to throw further, jump higher and punch harder! Although utilised as a sports-specific method of training, 'Plyos' presents a great challenge and not only benefits tremendously in terms of muscular fitness but also in the level of muscle contraction 'force' that you will be able to generate (motor skill), balance and co-ordination. It must also be noted here that thousands of exercises lower in intensity can be characterised as 'plyometrics' (Jumping Jacks, for example and anything which involves leaping, hopping or skipping is effectively a plyometric exercise).

Isometrics

Important: Useful exercises to include for the mini-workouts, however they should be avoided by anyone with high blood pressure.

This type of contraction involves no movement at the joint and is maintained in a static state (one example would be holding a Squat for a period of time until failure). The benefits in strength are considerable, however *only* at the angle of the joint.

Remember, in order to make gains in any area of physical fitness the principle of overload holds true. With muscular strength and endurance the muscle must work harder than it would do under normal circumstances to achieve gains. Of course this is all relative to the individual, but the benefits are consistent. Progression is achieved once the body has adapted to a workload (when a given task no longer presents any challenge) and resistance must be increased to continue making progress. In terms of bodyweight, this would mean altering the variation of an exercise to maintain a state of overload.

Frequency and Duration

If you are just starting out and you want to build strength, work out twice a week for 20 minutes using bodyweight exercises you can perform for 8-12 RM. As the body adapts to the workload, the exercise will become easier and at this point, progression may be made by graduating to a more challenging modification to remain within your target rep range for strength. If, however, you are working towards muscular endurance then you may want to work up to twenty-five reps on any given exercise – the frequency of workout can be increased as the body adapts even further.

The Core

The group of muscles running through your mid-section (trunk) is responsible for supporting your spine and keeping the body stable and balanced. As a whole, the core is often neglected and manifests in most people's workouts simply as 'Abs', but don't make this mistake! Your Rectus Abdominis constitute only one part of the jigsaw: it's main function is to flex the spine forwards. To develop core strength and stability, approach all muscles in the region in equal measure. The lower back is often a problem area for a great many people due to a lack of core conditioning. Achieving fitness in this area will not only act as a preventative measure against injury, but also improve posture, co-ordination, balance and stability.

Using your core to stabilise the body features heavily when performing exercise as you 'engage' the core to maintain correct form (technique) through a movement and the more conditioned your core becomes, the more efficiently you can execute physical tasks.

Without becoming too technical about it, the muscles involved are as follows:

Rectus abdominis (the long muscle extending along the front of the abdomen or in other words, the six-pack)

External Obliques (side and front of the abdomen)

Internal Obliques (directly below the External Obliques)

Erector spinae (three muscles situated in the middle of your lower back)

Transverse abdominis (a deep muscle, situated under the Internal Obliques).

We use these muscles daily to keep ourselves in a constant state of 'flexion' (upright). As we walk, bend, twist and reach, virtually every movement we make involves the core to certain extent and so to maintain and develop this area is paramount to enjoying a continuous injury- and pain-free life.

Core exercises feature as components of circuits and also as independent mini-workouts. In addition, our core muscles work by default in assisting, fixing and stabilising movement as we perform any exercise. There is often a debate as to how regularly we should exercise the core because the muscles in this area are not attached to bone and therefore respond differently to stimulus. Some believe in one day on and one day off as with any other muscle group, while others train the core every day. It is my opinion that as the core keeps us in a constant state of flexion it is designed to work on a daily basis and can be trained as such.

Motor Fitness

As I have hinted at earlier, motor fitness is skill-related and concerned with how the muscles perform in terms of balance, power, speed, co-ordination and reaction time. Direct work on motor fitness would be typically associated with enhancing sports performance, however the benefits of taking up regular exercise will improve your motor skills by default. On the whole, motor skills are based on a teacher-learner basis with reinforcement, feedback, motivation and demonstration playing an important role, however you can develop such skills by strictly following the exercise instructions in this book.

This becomes more pronounced as we enter the latter levels where plyometrics are used, which as well as being great fitness tools are specific to improving speed, power, balance and co-ordination. As your body becomes accustomed to repeated movements, the neuro-muscular system (connection between brain and muscles) is being educated and reinforced and over time, creates a more efficient relationship and higher performance levels.

Summary

If you have read this chapter as a sedentary or unfit person you will now understand the importance of starting off slowly and gradually building up your fitness levels. Use the methods contained within this chapter to build up your aerobic fitness by walking and progress to jogging. To increase anaerobic fitness, attempt easy variations until you can progress to the more difficult versions. Focus on maintaining the correct execution of exercises and monitor yourself properly: always warm up, cool down and definitely stretch afterwards.

Chapter Three
PRE- AND POST-WORKOUT PROCEDURE, FLEXIBILITY AND STRETCHING

Preparation for Workout
Warm-up (Five to Ten Minutes)

Preparing the body for exercise is vital as a preventative measure against injury and it is also instrumental in priming your 'readiness' for exertion. It is common practice to mobilise and pulse raise prior to exercising. 'Mobilising' consists of rhythmic movements of the joints and spine; it warms up synovial fluid around the membrane of the joints to assist in movement (synovial fluid is a thick fluid present in synovial joints such as the elbow, shoulder, knee, hip etc. Its function is to lubricate and assist in movement as well as shock absorb and nourish the joint). By increasing the heart rate ('pulse raise'), we increase body heat and blood flow to the muscles. This is important because our muscles need to be pliable to avoid injury and require up to 80 per cent of total blood flow to work efficiently at a high intensity, as opposed to just 15 per cent of total blood flow at rest. To pulse raise safely, always increase the intensity of exercise gradually.

Select warm-up exercises to complement or mimic those exercises that make up the main element of your workout. To save time, combine mobilising with your pulse raiser, as illustrated on page 34. Warm-up times vary from person to person, and are also dependent on factors such as an existing issue with joints or muscles, whether you are approaching warm up from being sedentary, and the environment (it can take longer to raise the body temperature if conditions are cold). Five minutes should be perfectly sufficient but if in doubt, listen to your body!

Should You Stretch As Part of the Warm-Up?

> **Important:** If you decide to prep-stretch after your initial pulse raiser, it is advisable to re-warm the body because your pulse rate will have dropped during stretching and therefore needs to be raised again. Some mini-workouts suggest a re-warm and, to avoid possible injury, this is advisable. If you have existing injuries, consult a specialist before stretching that particular joint. Listen to your body and stop if you feel pain: a good stretch causes mild discomfort, so make that distinction!

There remains much debate over the effectiveness of preparatory (or 'prep' stretches) before a workout. Prep stretches are traditionally static (without movement) and involve the exerciser stretching while standing (this saves time as the idea is to avoid the heart rate dropping). Typically these are held for six to eight seconds and in my opinion do not present long enough exposure to tension to sufficiently 'stretch' the muscle. In addition, there have also been studies to suggest that subjecting muscles to static stretch 'stress' prior to intense exercise could be detrimental to performance, that it also weakens the muscle and may offer no protection from injury. (see note at the end of this chapter) Opinions on sports physiology change on a regular basis, however, so if you are accustomed to prep stretching and find this effective there is nothing conclusive to suggest that you should stop now. Although I myself believe the benefits to be negligible, this is still an accepted recommendation.

Post-Workout
Cool Down: Maintenance and Developmental Stretches (Five to Ten Minutes)

'Cool Down' is performed after the main workout to steadily bring the body temperature and heart rate down and to continue the circulation of blood around the body. This helps to avoid fainting or dizziness, which can result from blood pooling in the large muscles of the legs when vigorous activity ceases suddenly. Abrupt cessation of exercise can also be harmful to the heart. As with the warm-up, similar rhythmical exercises are used gradually to safely decrease intensity and five minutes should be perfectly sufficient.

Post-exercise stretching is probably one of the most neglected areas of physical fitness yet it plays a vital role in keeping the body flexible and functioning at an optimum level. Stretching at this point is much more advantageous because the muscles are primed, pliable and contain more blood, so offering greater protection from injury and a safer 'environment' in which to develop a range of movement as well as aiding recovery from your workout and the elimination of waste products, including lactic acid.

There are many stretching terms, which can often lead to confusion: 'static' and 'passive' for example, are regularly used interchangeably. 'Static' stretching involves slowly assuming a position until the furthest point of a stretch where the muscle has reached its maximum length (the 'bite') and holding. 'Passive' stretching (referred to as 'static-passive' or 'relaxed' stretching) involves assuming a position and using an external force (some other part of your body or the help of a partner) to hold the stretch. Slow and relaxed, this stretch is ideal when cooling down. The following descriptions will help you distinguish between the various cool-down stretches.

Maintenance Stretches

Time held: Fifteen seconds
Held statically at 'the bite' for long enough to lengthen the muscle, maintain flexibility and prevent muscle soreness.

Developmental Stretches

Time held: Twenty-five to thirty seconds
Held statically at the 'bite' until the tension eases, at which point the muscle is stretched externally, further developing its length and the range of movement at the joint. Significant benefits may be achieved with small increments over time.
• Helps clear Lactic acid (waste product)

- Reduces D.O.M.S (Delayed Onset Muscle Soreness)
- Increases range of movement in the joints
- Reduces muscle tension
- Promotes blood to the muscles to aid workout recovery
- Improves muscular co-ordination, posture and sports performance.

Mobilising Joints

It is good practice to mobilise joints that will be employed in your main workout and in the case of the mini-workout, this means all the joints in the body. It takes only a short time (six to eight rotations of each joint is sufficient). Begin with smaller movements and gradually increase the range of movement as you go.

How to Mobilise and Pulse Raise

You may want to pay special attention to certain joints and include warm-up exercises closer to the mini-workout you are about to engage in. If, for example, the workout consists of press-up variations, you may prefer to do an easier modification in your warm-up (for example, kneeling press ups in preparation for full press ups).

Begin by slow walking with good posture (upright, shoulders back) while performing the movements that follow consecutively. The entire warm-up should take no more than three to five minutes:

Wrist Circles (six to eight rotations per wrist): Gently rotate each wrist in a circular motion.

Shoulder Shrugs (six to eight): Gently shrug both shoulders up to the ears and then back down again.

Shoulder Rolls (six to eight rotations per shoulder): With the arm bent, gently rotate each shoulder in turn.

Shoulder Circles (six to eight rotations per shoulder): Smoothly rotate each shoulder with a straight arm.

Now stop walking and perform each of the following exercises:

Ankle Circles (six to eight rotations per ankle): Stand with your feet hip-width apart and knees slightly bent. Extend one leg forward and off the ground, placing your weight on the standing leg while keeping a neutral spine (straight back) and using your arms as a counterweight for balance. Gently rotate the ankle, then repeat on the other side.

Hip Circles (six to eight rotations clockwise, then anti-clockwise): Stand with your feet a shoulder-width apart and knees slightly bent. Place your hands on your hips or out in front of you. Gently create a circular motion by transferring your weight forward to the side, back, then to the side again and forward: this should be a smooth rotation throughout.

Side Twists (four rotations each side to mobilise the middle back (thoracic spine): Stand with your feet hip-width apart and knees slightly bent, keeping a neutral spine (straight back). Hold your arms out in front and gently twist your torso to one side. Note: the entire lower body is fixed and only the upper body twists. Repeat four rotations alternating left and right and stopping between rotations.

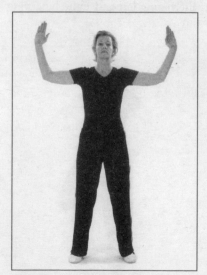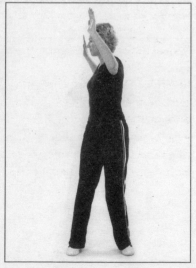

Side Twists

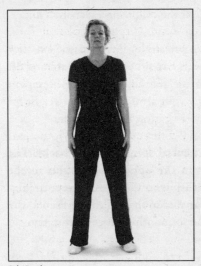
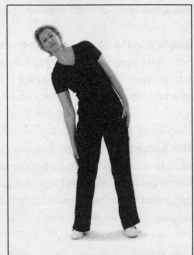

Side Bends

Side Bends (four rotations each side to mobilise the lower back (lumbar spine): Stand with your feet hip-width apart and knees slightly bent, keeping a neutral spine (straight back). Hold your arms by your sides and gently flex the body to one side, alternating left and right.

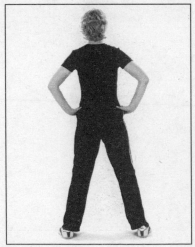
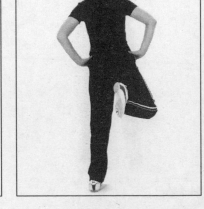

Flick Backs

Flick Backs (ten reps): Stand with your feet one-and-a-half shoulder-widths apart with the knees slightly bent, keeping a neutral spine (straight back). Place your hands on your hips or out in front. Now flick your heel back towards the glutes while transferring your weight to the standing leg. Repeat with your opposite heel. Continue this movement in a smooth, controlled manner.

Hop and Twist (ten rotations): Stand with your feet hip-width apart and knees slightly bent, keeping a neutral spine (straight back). The idea is to rotate your upper body in the opposite direction to the lower body, while looking ahead throughout the movement. Hop and rotate the legs and feet in one direction while simultaneously twisting the upper body in the opposite direction. This warm-up exercise is more dynamic and should be performed with a smooth, mid-tempo action.

Following this, I recommend you include a single exercise or several exercises that make up the main workout. For example:
High Knees Plus Skip, sixty to ninety seconds (see page 116)
Jumping Jacks, sixty to ninety seconds (see page 109)

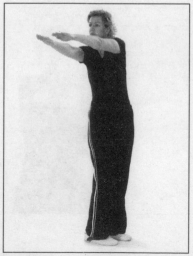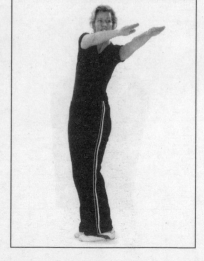

Hop and Twist

At this point you may opt to go straight into the selected mini-workout or proceed to preparatory stretches (see below). Once completed, re-warm the muscles with any rhythmical exercise (Jumping Jacks etc.)

For the re-warm and cool down, a simple light jog on the spot or High Knees for about five minutes or less is sufficient to raise or lower your pulse. A re-warm involves gradually raising the intensity, whereas a cool down is the opposite.

Stretches

Important: Select one stretch per body part.
Preparatory stretches are held for six to eight seconds (select only standing stretches to minimise time).
Maintenance stretches are held for fifteen to twenty seconds.
Developmental stretches are held for twenty-five to thirty seconds (as the tension eases, increase the range of motion).

Upper Body

Back of Upper Arm (Standing)   Front of Shoulder (Standing)

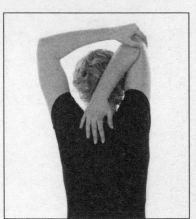
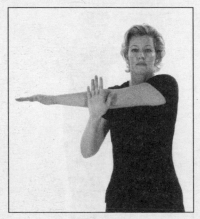

Chest (Standing)

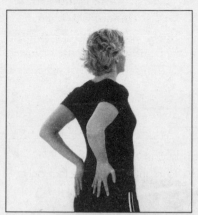

Upper Back (Standing)

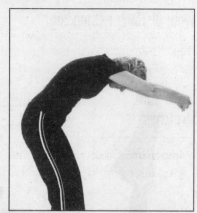

Forearm (Standing)

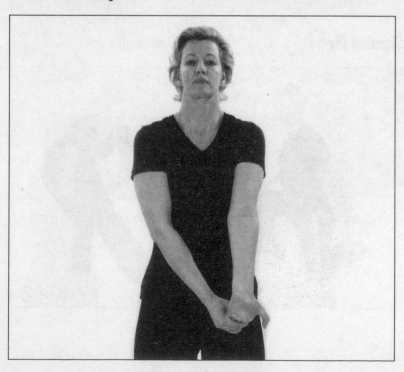

Lower Body

Front of Thigh I (Standing)

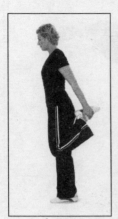

Front of Thigh II

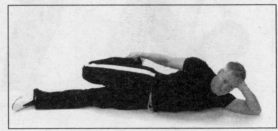

Front of Thigh III

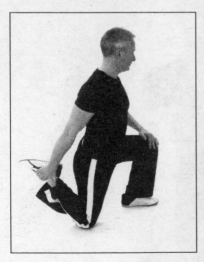

Back of Thigh I

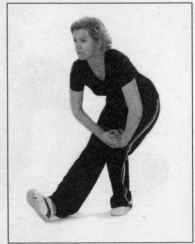

Back of Thigh II

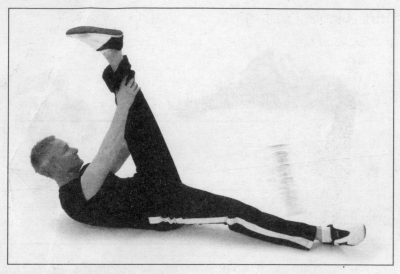

Inner Thigh

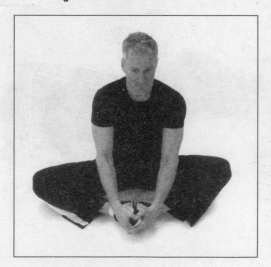

Calf (Standing)

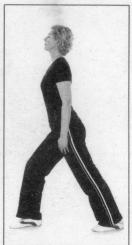

Glute

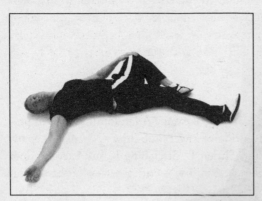

Lower Back I

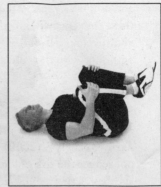

Lower Back II

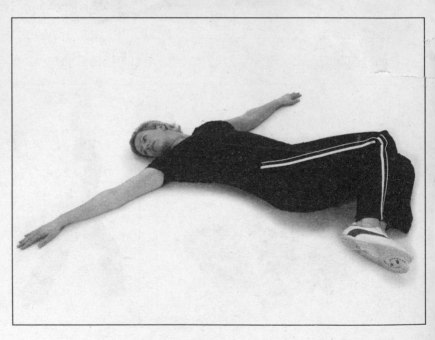

A good warm-up is vital to ensure you safely prepare the body for ensuing exercise. A good cool down and stretch is essential to maintain and improve muscle function and reduce muscle soreness. Excluding these elements will greatly reduce your level of performance and expose you to potential injury. If you want to continue to exercise safely and with longevity then always warm-up, cool down and stretch.

Notes

Pope, R.P., Herbert, R.D., and J.D. Kirwan. 'A randomised trial of pre-exercise stretching for prevention of lower limb injury', *Med. Sci. Sports Exerc.* 32:271–7 (2000) and Shrier, I. 'Stretching before exercise does not reduce the risk of local muscle injury: A critical review of the clinical and basic science literature', *Clinical J. Sports Med.* 9: 221–7 (1999).

Chapter Four

INDEX OF EXERCISES

Below is a complete list of all the exercises employed within this book. The smaller muscle group upper body exercises are listed first, followed by the larger muscle group lower body exercises; all core exercises are next in sequence, with the most challenging and more advanced Plyometric exercises listed last.

Upper Body Exercises

Floor Dip
Floor Extended Dip
Elevated Dip
Floor Dip with Extended Leg
Wall Press Up
Kneeling Press Up
Extended Kneeling Press Up
Splayed Leg Press Up
Standard Press Up
Dolphin Press Up
Standard Press Up with Raised Leg
T Press Up
Diamond Press Up
Spiderman Press Up
Hindu Press Up

One-handed Press Up
Hand to Forearm Press Up
Knuckle Press Up
Fingertip Press Up
Decline Press Up
Wide Press Up
Handstand Press Up

Lower Body Exercises

Standard Squat
Prisoner Squat
Bulgarian Squat
Wide Squat
One-leg Dead Lift
Pistol Squat
Calf Raises
Lunges
Reverse Lunges
Side-to-Side Squat
Squat Hold
Wall Squat

Core Exercises

Crunch
Oblique Crunch I
Oblique Crunch II
Reverse Crunch
Russian Twist
Windscreen Wiper
Bicycle
Seated-row Crunch
Oblique Seated-row Crunch
Raised Leg Crunch
Floor Bridge
V-Ups
Alternate V-Ups
Cheating V-Ups

Plank
Plank plus Raised Leg
Side Plank
Side Plank plus Raised Leg
Side Plank Rotator
Side Plank plus Twist
Side Bridge
Dorsal Raise
Superman

Plyometric Exercises

Extended Kneeling Plyo Press Up
Press Up with Hand Clap
Press Up with Chest Slap
Jumping Jacks
Mountain Climbers
Tuck Jumps
Jump Squats
Squat Kicks
Split Jumps
High Knees
High Knees plus Skip
Lunge Jumps
Ankle Jumps
Alternate Toe-Taps
Standard Burpee
Burpee (Non-Jump)
Burpee (Press Up)
Burpee (Tuck Jump)
Burpee (Long Jump)
One-handed Burpee

UPPER BODY EXERCISES

Floor Dip

The Floor Dip is used to develop muscular strength and endurance of
the upper body, with emphasis placed on the triceps.

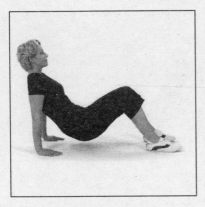
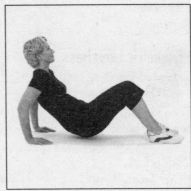

INSTRUCTIONS

(a) Extend your arms and keep them in line with your shoulders, palms
on the floor and fingers pointing forward. Your feet should be flat on
the floor, knees bent, with the lower legs perpendicular to the floor.

(b) Now lower the body by
bending at the elbows until you
almost touch the ground, then
immediately extend the elbows
and return to the start position
in a smooth and controlled
movement.

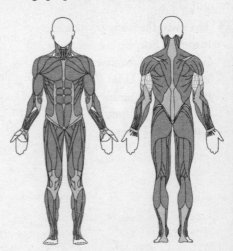

Targets: Backs of the arms
(Triceps Brachii)

Floor Extended Dip

The Floor Extended Dip is a progression from the Floor Dip (above) and used to develop muscular strength and endurance in the upper body, with emphasis placed on the backs of the arms.

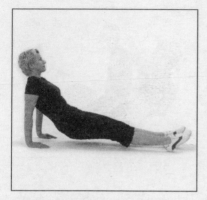
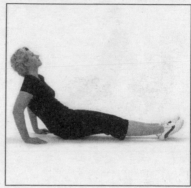

INSTRUCTIONS

(a) Extend your arms and keep them in line with your shoulders, palms on the floor and fingers pointing forward. Both legs should be extended in front, resting on your heels.

(b) Lower the body by bending at the elbows until you almost touch the ground then immediately extend the elbows and return to the start position in a smooth and controlled movement.

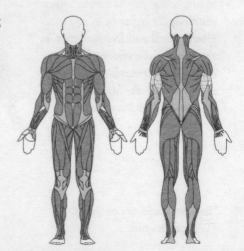

Targets: Backs of the arms
(Triceps Brachii)

Elevated Dip

The Elevated Dip is used to develop muscular strength and endurance in the upper body with emphasis placed on the backs of the arms; it represents a further level of difficulty to the Extended Floor Dip.

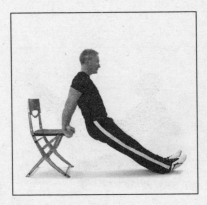 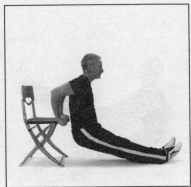

INSTRUCTIONS

(a) To achieve your starting position, sit on an elevated object such as a secure chair, with your hands placed on the edge of it, arms straight. Your legs should be straight with the heels on the floor. Now slide off the edge.

(b) Holding this position, lower the body by bending at the elbows until you feel a stretch in the chest and shoulders then immediately extend the elbows and return to the start position in a controlled movement.

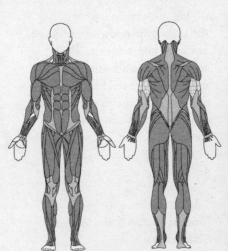

Targets: Backs of the arms
(Triceps Brachii)

Floor Dip with Extended Leg

The Floor Dip with Extended Leg is used to develop muscular strength and endurance in the upper body. Emphasis is simultaneously on the backs of the arms and abs as the leg is raised throughout so greatly beneficial to core strength and stability.

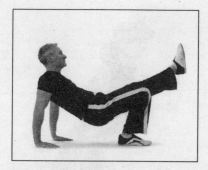 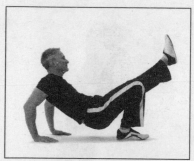

INSTRUCTIONS

(a) To achieve your starting position, extend the arms and keep them in line with your shoulders, palms towards the floor and fingers pointing forward. Your feet should be flat on the floor, knees bent, with the lower legs perpendicular to the floor. Straighten the left leg to point upwards in line with the angle of the right leg.

(b) Holding this position, lower the body by bending at the elbows until you almost touch the ground, then immediately extend the elbows and return to the start position. Pay careful attention to control the movement with your arms and core muscles. Alternate from one leg to another for the designated number of repetitions.

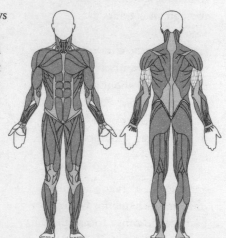

Targets: Backs of the arms (Triceps Brachii), Abs (Rectus Abdominis)

Wall Press Up

The Wall Press Up is used to develop muscular strength and endurance in the upper body. It represents the easiest press-up variation and will prepare you for progression onto the Kneeling Press Up (below).

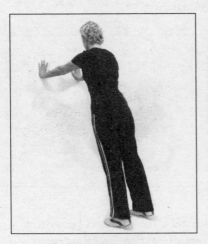 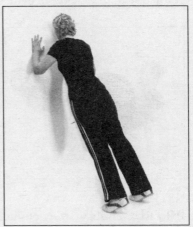

INSTRUCTIONS

(a) Stand facing a wall, approximately an arm's length away, and maintain a neutral stance. Raise your arms forward in line and slightly outside the shoulders, lean forward and place your hands on the wall to maintain a straight line through your spine.

(a) Bend at the elbows and slowly lower yourself towards the wall until about an inch away, then straighten your arms and slowly push back to the leaning position.

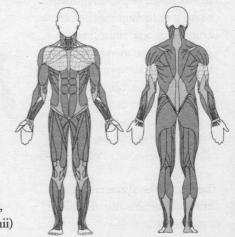

Targets: Chest (Pectorals), front of shoulders (Anterior Deltoids), backs of the arms (Triceps Brachii)

Kneeling Press Up

The Kneeling Press Up is used to develop muscular strength and endurance in the upper body and represents the progression from a Wall Press Up (above). Emphasis placed on the chest.

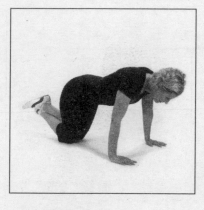 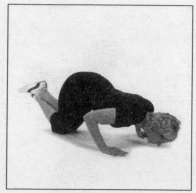

INSTRUCTIONS

(a) With your knees and feet resting on the floor, place your hands slightly wider than shoulder-width with the fingers facing forward. Aim to make a box shape with your arms, trunk, thighs and the floor.

(b) Now bend at your elbows and slowly lower your chest down to make a right angle with your arms (keep a straight line through your spine and avoid arching the back). Maintain a smooth rhythm throughout the exercise.

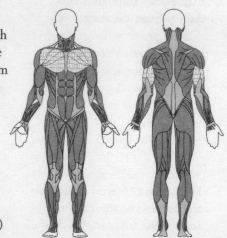

Targets: Chest (Pectorals), front of shoulders (Anterior Deltoids), backs of the arms (Triceps Brachii)

Extended Kneeling Press Up

The Extended Kneeling Press Up is used to develop muscular strength and endurance in the upper body and is a progression from the Kneeling Press Up (above). Emphasis placed on the chest.

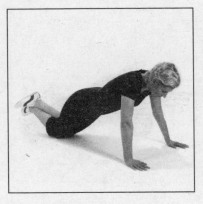 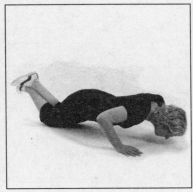

INSTRUCTIONS

(a) Support your body on your knees and cross your feet behind you. Now place your hands directly under and slightly wider than a shoulder-width apart maintaining a straight back.

(b) Lower your body by bending at the elbows until your chest nearly touches the floor (keep the body prone without allowing the hips to sag). Straighten your elbows to push back to start position.

Targets: Chest (Pectorals), front of shoulders (Anterior Deltoids) and the backs of the arms (Triceps Brachii)

Splayed Leg Press Up

The Splayed Leg Press Up is used to develop muscular strength and endurance in the upper body and represents a further progression to the Extended Kneeling Press Up (above). Emphasis is placed on the chest.

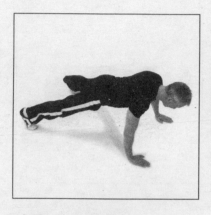 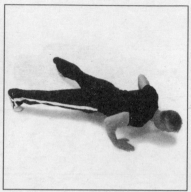

INSTRUCTIONS

(a) Support the body on the balls of your feet and place your hands directly under and slightly wider than a shoulder-width apart, while keeping your back in a straight line (prone position) from head to heel. Adjust your legs to a splayed position approximately one-and-a-half times hip-width apart.

(b) Lower your body by bending at the elbows until your chest nearly touches the floor (keep prone without allowing the hips to sag). Straighten your elbows to push back to start position.

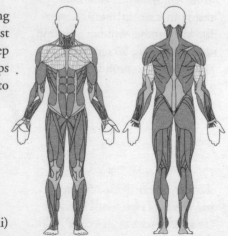

Targets: Chest (Pectorals), front of shoulders (Anterior Deltoids), backs of the arms (Triceps Brachii)

Standard Press Up

The Standard Press Up is used to develop muscular strength and endurance in the upper body with emphasis placed on the chest.

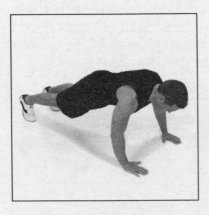 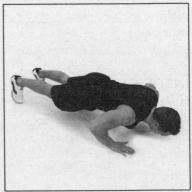

INSTRUCTIONS

(a) Support your body on the balls of the feet and place your hands directly under and slightly wider than a shoulder-width apart with your back in a straight line (prone position) from head to heel. Your feet can be together or hip-width apart.

(b) Lower your body by bending at the elbows until your chest nearly touches the floor. Keep the body prone without allowing the hips to sag. Straighten your elbows to push back to start position.

Targets: Chest (Pectorals), front of shoulders (Anterior Deltoids), backs of the arms (Triceps Brachii)

Dolphin Press Up

The Dolphin Press Up is used to develop muscular strength and endurance. It represents an interesting and easier alternative to a regular Press Up and is great preparation for building upper body strength to improve your Standard Press Up. The Abs are activated to great effect to maintain the integrity of the movement, thereby contributing to greater balance and core stability (strengthening of the mid-section).

INSTRUCTIONS

(a) Assume a plank position: rise onto the balls of your feet (held a hip-width apart) and stabilise your upper body with your elbows positioned below your shoulders, fingers clasped. Now maintain a straight line from head to heel. Contract your abdominals to prevent sagging in the midsection (or the opposite with your backside sticking up).

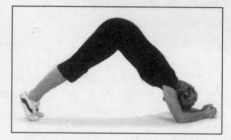

(b) Next, push with your forearms and raise your mid-section high in the air so your body forms an inverted 'V' (keep your head down and in line with your spine). Return to the starting position with a smooth movement.

Targets: Abs (Rectus Abdominis), chest (Pectorals), front of shoulders (Anterior Deltoids), backs of the arms (Triceps), back/upper and lower (Trapezius and Latissimus Dorsi)

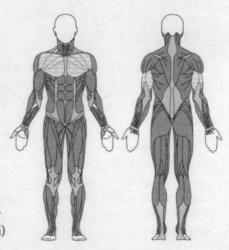

Standard Press Up with Raised Leg

The Raised Leg Press Up is used to develop muscular strength and endurance in the upper body. This variation represents a greater challenge than the Standard Press Up as the Abs are activated to great effect to maintain the raised leg throughout the movement, contributing to greater balance and core stability (strengthening of the mid-section).

INSTRUCTIONS

(a) Support your body on the balls of the feet and place your hands directly under and slightly wider than a shoulder-width apart, back in a straight line (prone position) from head to heel.

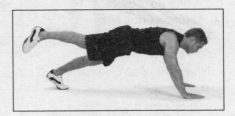

(b) Now lift one leg off the floor and lower your body by bending at the elbows until your chest nearly touches the floor, keeping the leg lifted throughout (keep the body prone without allowing the hips to sag by engaging the core muscles). Straighten your elbows to push back to start position. Complete the designated number of repetitions, then repeat on the other leg.

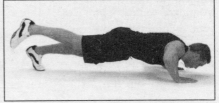

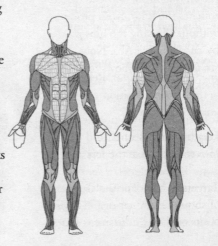

Targets: Chest (Pectorals), backs of the arms (Triceps Brachii), front of the shoulders (Anterior Deltoids), Abs (Rectus Abdominis)

T Press Up

The T Press Up is used to develop muscular strength and endurance in the upper body and has the added benefit of improving balance and co-ordination. Emphasis placed on the chest.

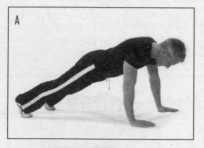

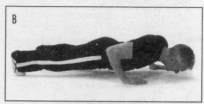

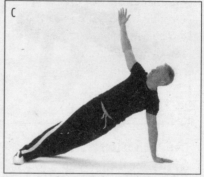

INSTRUCTIONS

(a) Support your body on the balls of the feet and place your hands directly under and slightly wider than a shoulder-width apart, back in a straight line (prone position) from head to toe.

(b) Lower your body by bending at the elbows until your chest nearly touches the floor. Keep prone without allowing the hips to sag by engaging the Abs. Now straighten your elbows to push back to start position.

(c) From the start position and keeping this as one fluid movement, raise the left arm to

Targets: Chest (Pectorals), front of shoulders (Anterior Deltoids), backs of the arms (Triceps Brachii)

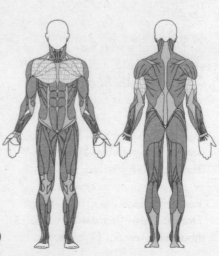

form a T-shape. Return the arm to the start position, perform another Press Up and form a T-shape with your right arm. Alternate for the designated amount of repetitions and maintain a smooth rhythm throughout.

Diamond Press Up

The Diamond Press Up is used to develop muscular strength and endurance in the upper body with emphasis placed on the triceps.

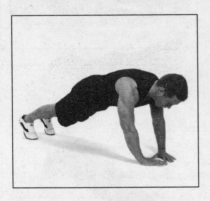
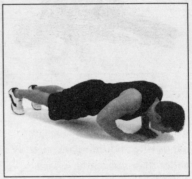

INSTRUCTIONS

(a) Assume the press up (prone) position with your body in a straight line from head to toe (hands set in line with your shoulders, arms straight).

(b) Now bring your hands together to create a diamond shape with index fingers and thumbs. Lower yourself towards the floor until your chest touches your hands (keep your back straight throughout). Push back to starting position.

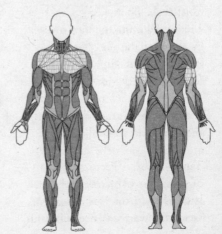

Targets: Backs of the arms (Triceps Brachii), chest (Pectorals), front of shoulders (Anterior Deltoids)

Spiderman Press Up

The Spiderman Press Up is used to develop muscular strength and endurance in the upper body. Throughout the movement, the action of the leg activates the abs, contributing to greater balance, co-ordination and core stability (strengthening of the mid-section). Emphasis is placed on the chest.

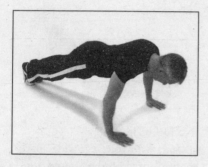 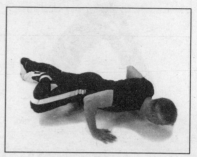

INSTRUCTIONS

(a) Start by assuming a press-up position: support your body on the balls of the feet and place your hands directly under and slightly wider than a shoulder-width apart, with your back in a straight line (prone position) from head to heel.

(b) When lowering yourself simultaneously, bend your knee to bring your right leg beside you so that the thigh approaches your torso and the knee almost touches your elbow. As you press up, reverse the leg action back to the starting position. Repeat the same process with your left leg then alternate from left to right for the designated amount of repetitions in a slow and controlled movement.

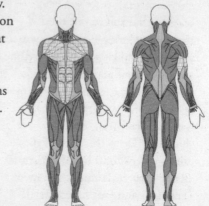

Targets: Chest (Pectorals), front of shoulders (Anterior Deltoids), back of the arms (Triceps Brachii), Abs (Rectus Abdominis).

Hindu Press Up

The Hindu Press Up is used to develop muscular strength and endurance, stamina and flexibility of the joints. This movement activates the abs, contributing to greater balance, co-ordination and core stability (strengthening of the mid-section). Emphasis is placed on the upper body.

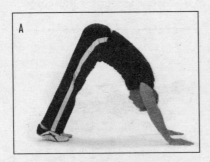

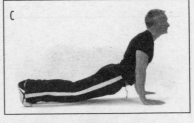

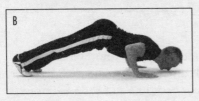

INSTRUCTIONS

(a) Start with your legs wide apart, hands planted on the ground and the midsection raised high in the air so your body forms an inverted 'V' (be sure to keep your head down so you don't strain your neck).

(b) Swoop down so your nose almost touches the floor, followed by the chin and chest in a controlled and paced way. Maintain control so you end up in the 'down' position, with your back straight.

(c) Continue this in one fluid movement. Swing forward so you arch your back and look up to the ceiling, with your arms and back extended. Reverse action back to start position.

Targets: Chest (Pectorals), shoulders (Deltoids), back of the arms (Triceps Brachii), Abs (Rectus Abdominis), back/upper and lower (Trapezius and Latissimus Dorsi)

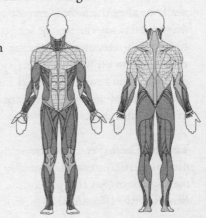

One-handed Press Up

The One-Handed Press Up is used to develop muscular strength and endurance in the upper body. This variation of the Press Up represents a greater challenge to the Standard Press Up (page 56) with emphasis placed on the shoulder and back of the arm individually. The core muscles are engaged to greater effect to assist throughout the movement.

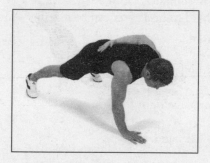
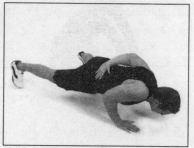

INSTRUCTIONS

(a) Support your body on the balls of the feet and place your hands directly under and slightly wider than a shoulder-width apart; keep your back in a straight line (prone position) from head to heel.

(b) Now widen the distance between your feet to stabilise approximately one-and-a-half times shoulder-width. Place your left arm behind your back then lower the body by bending at the elbow until your chest nearly touches the floor. Keep prone without allowing the hips to sag by engaging the core muscles. Straighten your elbow to push back to start position. Complete the designated number of repetitions and then repeat with the other arm.

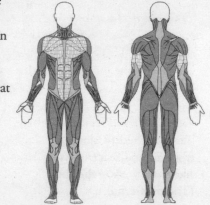

Targets: Chest (Pectorals), back of the arms (Triceps Brachii), front of the shoulders (Anterior Deltoids), Abs (Rectus Abdominis)

Hand to Forearm Press Up

The Hand to Forearm Press Up is used to develop muscular strength and endurance in the upper body with emphasis placed on the chest.

INSTRUCTIONS

(a) Support your body on the balls of your feet and place your hands directly under and slightly wider than shoulder-width apart, back in a straight line (prone position) from head to heel. Feet can be together or hip-width apart.

(b) Lower your body by dropping onto left forearm.

(c) Followed quickly by dropping onto the right forearm.

(d) Extend the left arm to return to left hand.

(e) Extend the right arm back to right hand and start position, this constitutes one repetition. Keep the body prone without allowing the hips to sag throughout. This exercise should be performed under control at a medium to fast tempo.

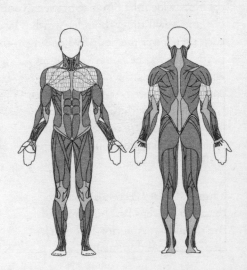

Targets: Chest (Pectorals), front of shoulders (Anterior Deltoids), back of the arms (Triceps Brachii)

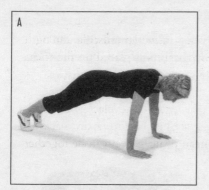

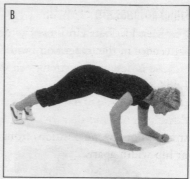

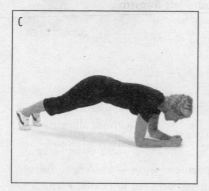

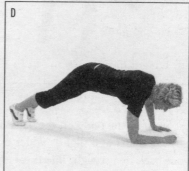

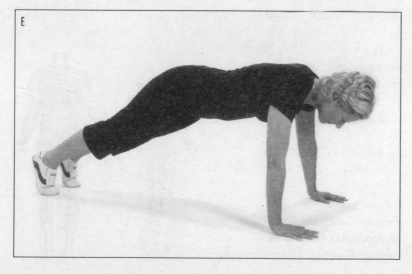

Knuckle Press Up

The Knuckle Press Up is used to develop muscular strength and endurance in the upper body with emphasis placed on the chest. This exercise is designed to strengthen the wrists and forearm muscles.

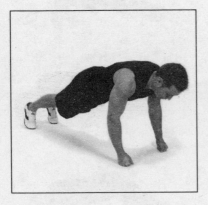 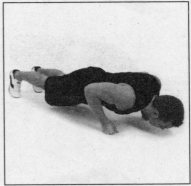

INSTRUCTION

(a) Support the body on the balls of your feet and place your hands directly under and slightly wider than a shoulder-width apart; keep your back in a straight line (prone position) from head to heel. Adjust your hand placement to support yourself on your knuckles, keeping the wrists straight throughout the exercise.

(b) Lower your body by bending at the elbows until your chest nearly touches the floor. Keep the body prone without allowing the hips to sag by engaging your core muscles. Now straighten your elbows to push back to start position.

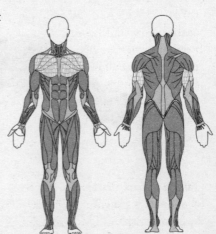

Targets: Chest (Pectorals), front of shoulders (Anterior Deltoids), back of the arms (Triceps Brachii)

Fingertip Press Up

The Fingertip Press Up is used to develop muscular strength and endurance in the upper body with emphasis on the chest. This exercise is designed to strengthen the muscles of the hand.

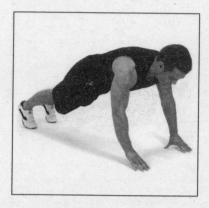
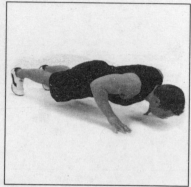

INSTRUCTIONS

(a) Support your body on the balls of the feet and place your hands directly under and slightly wider than a shoulder-width apart; keep your back in a straight line (prone position) from head to heel. Now rise up onto your fingertips and remain on them throughout the exercise.

(b) Lower your body by bending at the elbows until your chest nearly touches the floor (keep prone without allowing the hips to sag by engaging the core muscles). Straighten your elbows to push back to start position.

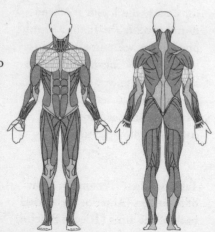

Targets: Chest (Pectorals), front of shoulders (Anterior Deltoids), back of the arms (Triceps Brachii)

Decline Press Up

The Decline Press Up is used to develop muscular strength and endurance with emphasis placed on the upper chest.

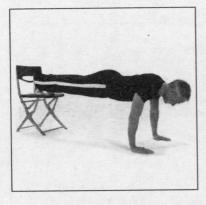
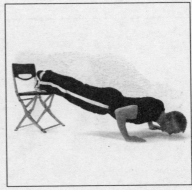

INSTRUCTIONS

(a) Support your body by placing the balls of your feet on an elevated object (chair etc – make sure it's stable) and place your hands on the floor directly under and slightly wider than shoulder-width apart, back in a straight line (prone position) from head to heel. Ensure your balance is secure.

(b) Lower your body by bending the elbows until your forehead nearly touches the floor. Keep the body prone without allowing the hips to sag by engaging the core muscles. Straighten your elbows to push back to start position. This should be a smooth and controlled movement.

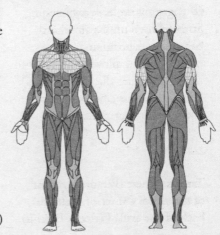

Targets: Chest (Pectorals), front of shoulders (Anterior Deltoids), back of the arms (Triceps Brachii)

Wide Press Up

The Wide Press Up is used to develop muscular strength and endurance in the upper body with emphasis placed on the shoulders.

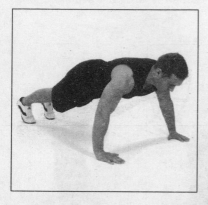 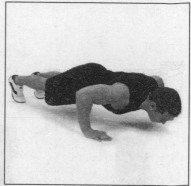

INSTRUCTIONS

(a) Support your body on the balls of the feet and place your hands in line, but wider than a shoulder-width apart; keep your back in a straight line (prone position) from head to heel. Feet can be together or a hip-width apart.

(b) Now lower your body by bending at the elbows until your chest nearly touches the floor. Keep prone without allowing the hips to sag by engaging the core muscles. Straighten your elbows to push back to start position.

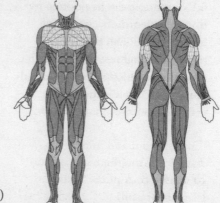

Targets: Chest (Pectorals), front of shoulders (Anterior Deltoids), back of the arms (Triceps Brachii)

Handstand Press Up

The Handstand Press Up is used to develop muscular strength and endurance in the upper body with emphasis placed on the shoulders. This is an advanced exercise and so caution is advised when attempting it for the first time.

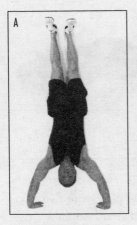
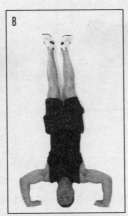
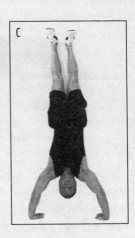

INSTRUCTIONS

(a) Assume a handstand position up against the wall with your arms fully extended and hands slightly wider than a shoulder-width apart.

(b) Now lower yourself until your head touches the floor.

(c) Return to the start position by driving your arms back into full extension. **NB This should not be attempted if you are a beginner. This exercise requires considerable strength, balance and co-ordination and is included as a Level 3 exercise only.**

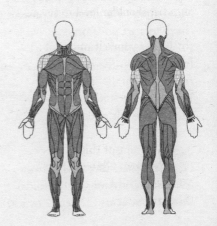

Targets: Front and middle of shoulders (Anterior and Lateral Deltoids), back of the arms (Triceps Brachii)

LOWER BODY EXERCISES

Standard Squat

The Standard Squat is used to develop muscular strength and
endurance in the lower body and represents one of the most complete
lower body exercises as it uses virtually all the leg muscles. Emphasis
placed on the front of the thighs.

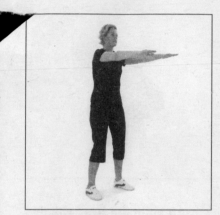 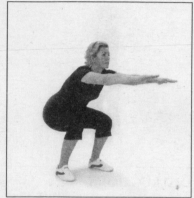

INSTRUCTIONS

(a) Stand with your feet slightly wider than a hip-width apart, with the
toes slightly turned out. Keep a neutral spine (straight back), knees
slightly bent and the arms extended
ahead at shoulder level to stabilise.

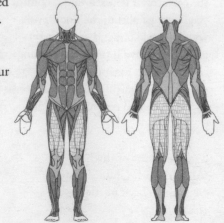

(b) Lower yourself under control
by bending at the knees until your
thighs are parallel to the floor.
Push your backside out, contract
the abdominals and engage the

Targets: Front of thighs
(Quadriceps), Glutes (Gluteus
Maximus), back of the legs
(Hamstrings)

lower back to stabilise (avoid your knees coming out over the toes).
Extend at the knees to return to the starting position. Perform in a
smooth and controlled action.

Prisoner Squat

The Prisoner Squat is used to develop muscular strength and endurance
in the lower body and represents a slightly more difficult variation on the
Standard Squat (above). Emphasis is placed on the front of the thighs.

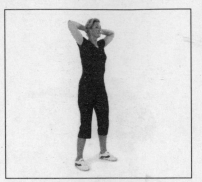
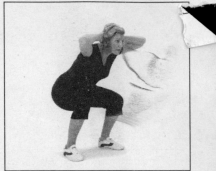

INSTRUCTIONS
(a) Stand with your feet slightly wider than a hip-width apart with the
toes just turned out. Keep a neutral spine (straight back), knees slightly
bent and place your palms behind your head, elbows raised.

(b) Now lower yourself under control by bending at the knees until your
thighs are parallel to the floor. Push
your backside out and contract the
abdominals (avoid the knees coming
over the toes). Extend at the knees to
return to the starting position. Perform
in a smooth and controlled action.

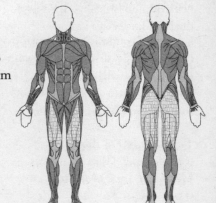

Targets: Front of thighs
(Quadriceps), Glutes (Gluteus
Maximus), back of the legs
(Hamstrings)

Bulgarian Squat

The Bulgarian Squat is used to develop muscular strength and endurance in the lower body and represents a further level of difficulty to the Standard Squat (page 71), with added benefits in balance and co-ordination. Emphasis is placed on the front of the thighs.

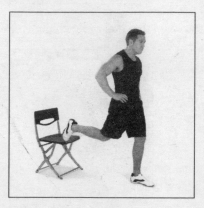 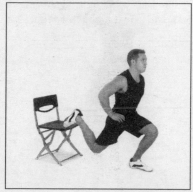

INSTRUCTIONS

(a) Extend the left leg back behind you and place the ball of your foot on an elevated object such as a chair (make sure this is secure) while supporting yourself on your right leg, placed a few feet ahead.

(b) Now lower yourself towards the floor into a lunge position, keeping the body straight and maintaining a neutral spine (straight back). Ensure the right knee stays in line with the heel and does not come over the toe. Once the thigh is parallel to the floor, push back to the start position. Swap legs to repeat the exercise. Perform in a smooth and controlled action.

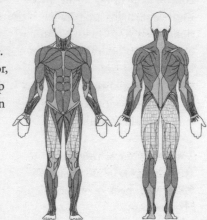

Targets: Front of thighs (Quadriceps), Glutes (Gluteus Maximus), back of the legs (Hamstrings)

Wide Squat

The Wide Squat is used to develop muscular strength and endurance in the lower body. Emphasis is placed on the front of the thighs.

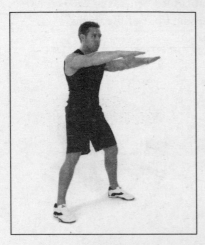
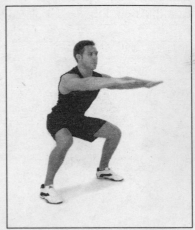

INSTRUCTIONS

(a) Stand with your feet approximately a double hip-width apart, with the toes slightly turned out. Keep a neutral spine (straight back), knees slightly bent and arms extended ahead at shoulder level to stabilise.

(b) Now lower yourself under control by bending at the knees until your thighs are parallel to the floor. Push your backside out and contract the abdominals (avoid the knees coming over the toes). Extend at the knees to return to the starting position. Perform in a smooth and controlled action.

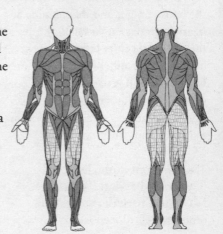

Targets: Front of thighs (Quadriceps), Glutes (Gluteus Maximus), back of the legs (Hamstrings)

One-Leg Dead Lift

The One-Leg Dead Lift is used to develop muscular strength and endurance of the lower body with emphasis placed on the back of the legs.

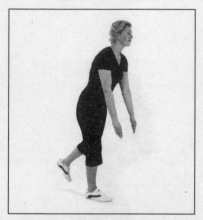 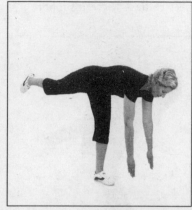

INSTRUCTIONS

(a) Stand with your feet a hip-width apart and the knees slightly bent while maintaining a neutral spine (straight back). Bend forward from the waist and allow your arms to drop freely towards the floor, simultaneously lifting one leg off the floor until it is in line with your body and parallel to the floor.

(b) Return the leg to the start position. Once the repetitions are complete, repeat with the opposite leg. Perform in a smooth and controlled action.

Targets: Back of legs (Hamstrings), Glutes (Gluteus Maximus), front of thighs (Quadriceps)

Pistol Squat

The Pistol Squat is used to develop muscular strength and endurance in the lower body. Emphasis is placed on the front of the thighs. This is an extremely challenging exercise and requires considerable practice to master. Once it becomes easier, you can attempt the exercise freestanding, without support.

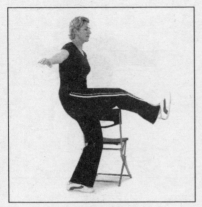 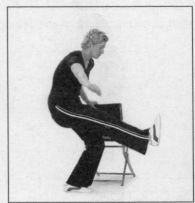

INSTRUCTIONS

(a) Stand with your feet approximately a shoulder-width apart with the toes slightly turned out. Keep a neutral spine (straight back), with your knees slightly bent and the arms extended at each side to stabilise.

(b) Raise one foot and extend forward. Now push your backside out, contract the abdominals and lower yourself under control by bending at the knee until your thigh is parallel to the floor. Push hard with your Glutes,

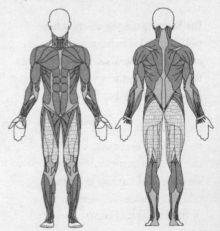

Targets: Front of the thighs (Quadriceps), Glutes (Gluteus Maximus), back of the legs (Hamstrings)

Hamstrings and Quadriceps to return to the start position. This is a slow, controlled and highly focused exercise.

NB This should not be attempted if you are a beginner. This exercise requires considerable strength, balance and co-ordination and is included as a Level 3 exercise only.

Calf Raises

The Calf Raise is used to develop muscular strength and endurance with emphasis placed on the calf muscles.

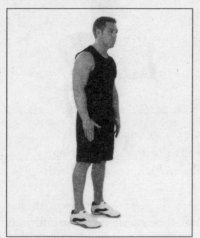

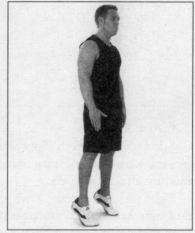

INSTRUCTIONS

(a) Stand with your feet a hip-width apart, keeping a neutral spine (straight back) and your legs straight, with the knees locked and hands by your sides.

(b) Smoothly rise up onto your toes to full extension and back to the starting position. Perform in a smooth and controlled action.

Targets: Calves (Gastrocnemius)

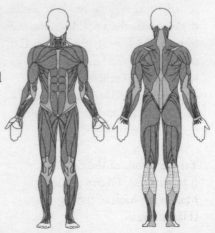

Lunges

Lunges are used to develop muscular strength and endurance in the lower body, with added benefits in balance and co-ordination. Emphasis is placed on the front of the thighs.

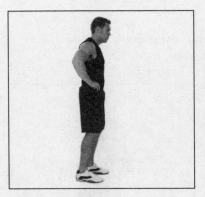

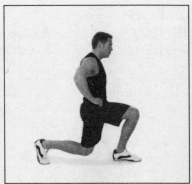

INSTRUCTIONS

(a) Stand with your feet a hip-width apart, with the toes facing forward. Keep a neutral spine (straight back), knees slightly bent and your arms by your side.

(b) Now take a long, comfortable stride forward (about 90cm/3ft). Bend the knee and lower yourself towards the floor, keeping the body straight and maintaining a straight back (ensure the knee does not come over the toe). To return to the start position, drive off the front foot and repeat the movement with the opposite leg. Perform in a smooth and controlled action.

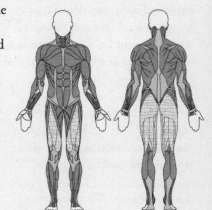

Targets: Front of thighs (Quadriceps), Glutes (Gluteus Maximus), back of the legs (Hamstrings)

Reverse Lunges

The Reverse Lunge is used to develop muscular strength and
endurance in the lower body, with added benefits in balance and
co-ordination. Emphasis is placed on the front of the thighs.

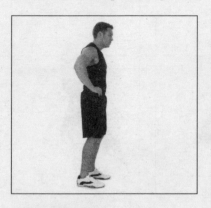 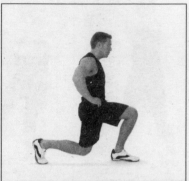

INSTRUCTIONS

(a) Stand with your feet a hip-width apart and your toes facing
forward. Keep a neutral spine (straight back), knees slightly bent
and arms by your sides.

(b) Take a long comfortable stride backwards (about 9ocm/3ft). Bend
the knee and lower yourself towards the floor, keeping the body
straight and maintaining a straight
back (ensure the standing knee does
not come over the toe). To return to
the start position, drive off the front
foot and repeat this movement with
the opposite leg. Perform in a
smooth and controlled action.

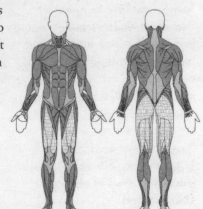

Targets: Front of thighs
(Quadriceps), Glutes (Gluteus
Maximus), back of the legs
(Hamstrings)

Side-to-Side Squat

The Side-to-Side Squat is used to develop muscular strength and
endurance in the lower body. Emphasis is placed on the front of the thighs.

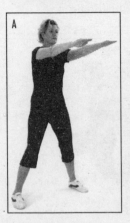
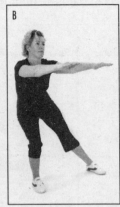
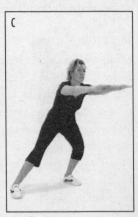

INSTRUCTIONS

(a) Stand with your feet one and a half times shoulder-width apart, with
the toes slightly turned out. Keep a neutral spine (straight back), knees
slightly bent and your arms extended ahead at shoulder level to stabilise.

(b) Lower yourself under control by bending one knee until your thigh
is parallel to the floor (the
opposite leg straightens as your
weight is shifted to one side).
Now push your backside out and
contract the abdominals (avoid
the knees coming over the toes).

(c) Reverse this action and repeat
with opposite leg.

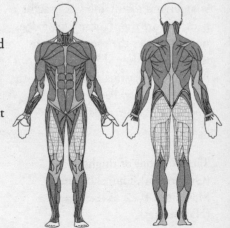

Targets: Front of thighs
(Quadriceps), Glutes (Gluteus
Maximus), back of the legs
(Hamstrings)

Squat Hold

The Squat Hold is used for muscular strength and endurance. As in all Isometric exercises, the development of strength is improved at the angle of the joint as the hold is maintained statically for a time.

INSTRUCTIONS

Stand with your feet somewhat wider than hip-width apart with toes slightly turned out. Keep a neutral spine, knees slightly bent and arms extended ahead at shoulder level to `stabilise you. Lower yourself under control by bending the knees until your thighs are parallel with floor. Push your backside out and contract the abdominals, avoid the knees coming over the toes. Hold this position without any movement for the designated period of time, usually between 30-60 seconds.

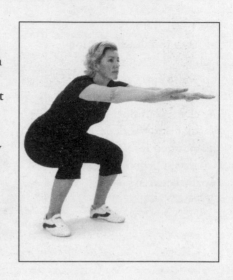

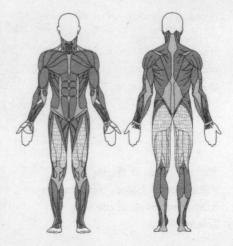

Targets: Front of thighs (Quadriceps) Glutes (Gluteus Maximus), Back of the legs (Hamstrings)

Wall Squat

The Wall Squat is used for muscular strength and endurance. As in all Isometric exercises, the development of strength is improved at the angle of the joint as the hold is maintained statically for a time.

INSTRUCTIONS
(a) Assume a seated position against a wall with your feet a hip-width apart and hands either on the wall or across the chest; your thighs should be parallel to the floor. Hold this position for the designated period of time, usually between 30–60 seconds.

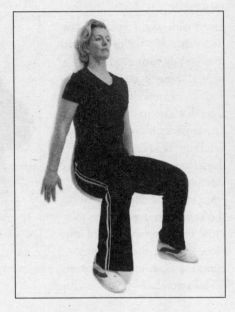

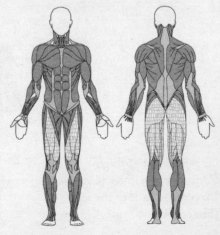

Targets: Front of thighs (Quadriceps) Glutes (Gluteus Maximus), Back of the legs (Hamstrings)

CORE EXERCISES

Crunch

The Crunch is used to develop muscular strength and endurance of the core. Emphasis is placed on the Abs.

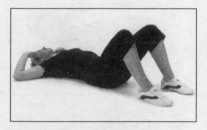 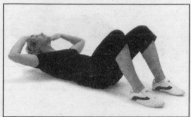

INSTRUCTIONS

(a) Lie on your back with your knees bent and your hips and feet flat on the floor. Place your hands behind or beside your neck, or across your chest.

(b) Now contract your Abs while lifting your shoulder blades off the floor and curling the shoulders towards your pelvis. To avoid injury, do not put any pressure on your neck throughout this movement: it should be a controlled, squeezing action.

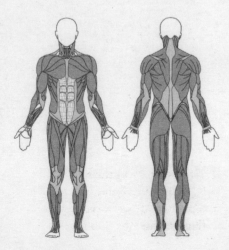

Targets: Abs (Rectus Abdominis)

Oblique Crunch I

The Oblique Crunch is used to develop muscular strength and endurance of the core. Emphasis placed on the Obliques (Side Abs).

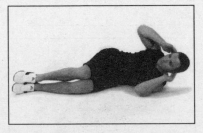 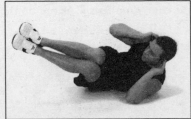

INSTRUCTIONS

(a) Lie sideways on the floor, supporting yourself on your right elbow, with your hands behind your head. Keep your legs flat on the floor, with the knees bent.

(b) Raise and twist the torso towards the hips (using the oblique/inner mid-section of torso), while simultaneously lifting the knees a few inches off the floor and draw them in the same direction. Perform this movement in a slow and controlled manner, feeling the squeeze, and return to the start position.

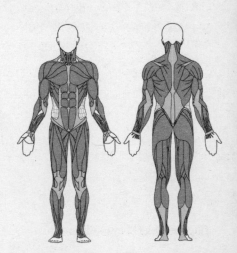

Targets: Side Abs (Obliques)

Oblique Crunch II

Like the previous exercise, the Oblique Crunch is used to develop
muscular strength and endurance of the core. Emphasis placed on
the Obliques (Side Abs).

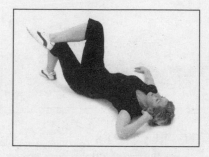
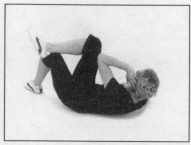

INSTRUCTIONS

(a) Lie on your back, with your knees bent and your hips and feet flat
on the floor. Place your hands behind your neck or at the sides of your
head and place your right foot across your left knee.

(b) Now contract your Abs while lifting your back off the floor, curling
your left shoulder and elbow towards your right knee. To avoid injury,
do not put any pressure on your neck throughout this movement –
this should be a controlled, squeezing action. Perform the designated
number of repetitions, then switch
legs and repeat on the other side.

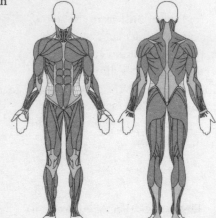

Targets: Side Abs (Obliques)

Reverse Crunch

The Reverse Crunch is used to develop muscular strength and endurance of the core. Emphasis placed on the Abs.

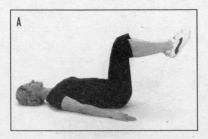

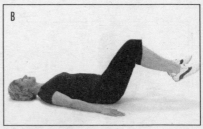

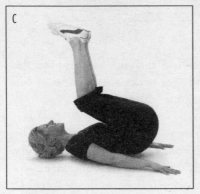

INSTRUCTIONS

(a) Lie flat on the floor, with your arms by your side and the palms facing down. Hold your knees at 90 degrees.

(b) Now raise your hips off the floor and bring the knees towards the chest by contracting the abdominals (use your hands to stabilise the movement).

(c) Return the legs to the start position under control (avoid using momentum and use only the abdominals throughout the movement). Perform in a slow and controlled manner, feeling the squeeze and returning to the start position.

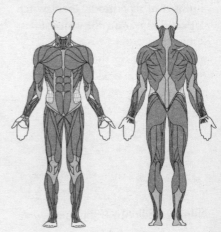

Targets: Abs (Rectus Abdominis)

Russian Twist

The Russian Twist is used to develop muscular strength and endurance. This exercise is especially good at building core stability throughout the torso.

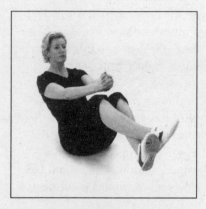 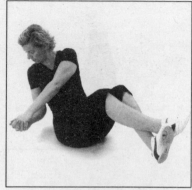

INSTRUCTIONS

(a) Start by sitting on your backside and draw your knees in towards your chest, keeping your feet off the floor and hands clasped in front.

(b) Simultaneously twist your upper and lower body in opposite directions. Keep your head in line with the spine when twisting the upper body and knees together, with your feet off the ground in the opposite direction. Maintain a smooth and controlled action from side to side without pausing.

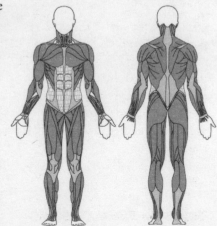

Targets: Abs (Rectus Abdominis), Side Abs (Obliques)

Windscreen Wiper

The Windscreen Wiper is used to develop muscular strength and endurance of the core. Emphasis is placed on the Abs.

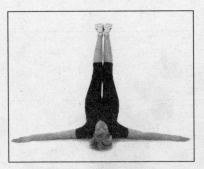

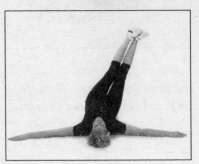

INSTRUCTIONS

(a) Lie on your back with your arms extended to one side. Now raise your legs upwards with the knees slightly bent.

(b) Lower your legs to one side until the thigh closest to the floor touches it. Raise and lower the legs to the opposite side in a 'wiper' motion. This should be a slow and controlled movement.

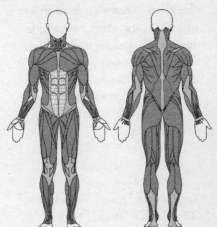

Targets: Abs (Rectus Abdominus)

Bicycle Crunch

The Bicycle Crunch is used to develop muscular strength and endurance of the core. Emphasis is placed on the abs.

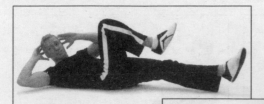

INSTRUCTIONS

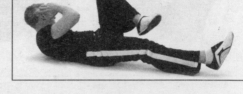

(a) Lie on your back and place your palms behind your head. Now bring the knees towards the chest and lift your shoulder blades off the ground (refrain from placing stress on the neck to avoid injury).

(b) Straighten the left leg while turning your torso to the right and bring your left elbow towards the right knee. Continue by doing the opposite action: right elbow to left knee. The idea is to create a smooth and rhythmic pedalling action. Ensure you maintain good form throughout: contract the abdominals and fully extend the trailing leg as you alternate sides.

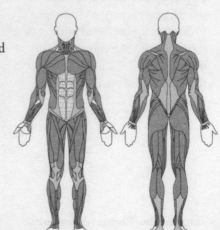

Targets: Abs (Rectus Abdominis)

Seated Row Crunch

The Seated Row Crunch is used to develop muscular strength and
endurance of the core. Emphasis placed on the abs.

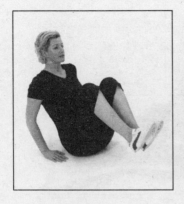

INSTRUCTIONS

(a) Start by sitting on your backside and draw your knees in towards
your chest, keeping your feet off the floor. Now prop yourself up using
your arms with hands facing forward.

(b) Extend both legs forward until straight while rocking backwards.
Continue this 'rowing' action for the prescribed repetitions. To make
the exercise more of a challenge,
perform it unsupported with your
hands across your chest. Perform
in a controlled manner, feeling
the squeeze and return to the
start position.

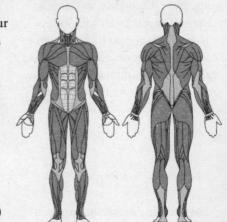

Targets: Abs (Rectus Abdominis)

Oblique Seated Row Crunch

The Oblique Seated Row Crunch is used to develop muscular strength and endurance of the core. Emphasis placed on the Side Abs (Obliques).

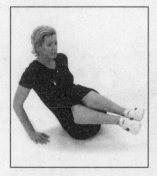

INSTRUCTIONS

(a) Start by sitting on your backside and prop yourself up using your arms with hands facing forward. Now bring your knees together and twist the torso with the knees pointing to the left and then raise towards the chest to squeeze the Obliques.

(b) Extend both legs forward until straight while rocking backwards, then bring the knees back to the chest and continue this 'rowing' action for the prescribed repetitions. Change sides and repeat.

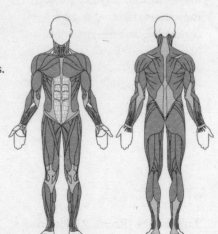

Targets: Side Abs (Obliques)

Raised Leg Crunch

The Raised Leg Crunch is used to develop muscular strength and endurance of the core and represents a more intense variation to the regular crunch.

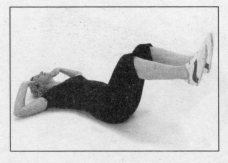
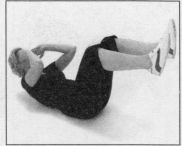

INSTRUCTIONS

(a) Lie on your back with your knees bent, hips and feet flat on the floor. Now raise your legs into a right-angle position. Place your hands behind or beside your neck, or across your chest.

(b) Contract your Abs while lifting your shoulder blades off the floor and curling your shoulders towards your pelvis (to avoid injury, do not put any pressure on your neck throughout this movement). This should be a controlled, squeezing action.

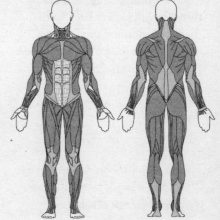

Targets: Abs (Rectus Abdominis)

Floor Bridge

The Floor Bridge is used to develop muscular strength and endurance of the core and lower body.

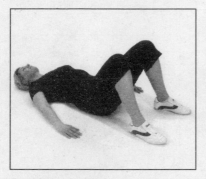 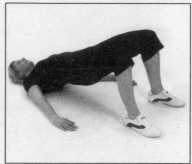

INSTRUCTIONS

(a) Lie on your back with legs bent and feet flat on the floor.

(b) Relax head and shoulders as you raise the hips, holding for 2-3 seconds at the top of the lift, squeeze the glutes then slowly lower the hips without touching the ground and repeat for repetitions.

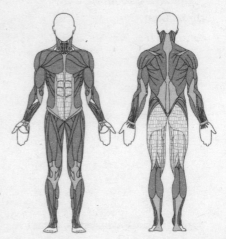

Targets: Abs (Rectus Abdominis), Glutes (Gluteus Maximus), back of the legs (Hamstrings)

V-Ups

Use V-Ups to develop muscular strength and endurance of the core.
Emphasis is placed on the Abs.

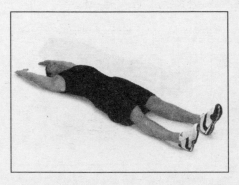 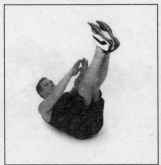

INSTRUCTIONS

(a) Start by lying on your back (supine) legs straight and arms above
your head.

(b) Keeping your legs and arms straight simultaneously bring them
together while raising your torso, then reverse the action back to
starting position with your back flat on the floor before starting a
further repetition. Let the abdominal muscles work dynamically and
maintain a smooth rhythm
throughout.

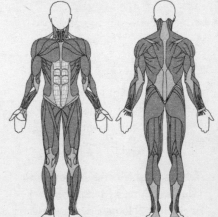

Targets: Abs (Rectus Abdominis)

Alternate V-Ups

Alternate V-Ups are used to develop muscular strength and endurance of the core; they are similar in difficulty to V-Ups but involve added rotation of the core muscles. Emphasis is placed on the Abs.

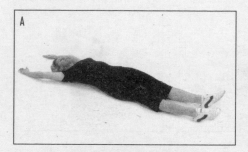

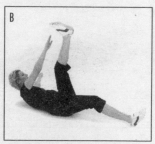

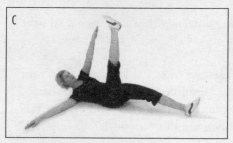

INSTRUCTIONS
(a) Start by lying on your back (supine), legs straight and arms above your head.

(b) Simultaneously bring your left leg to right hand while raising your torso

(keep limbs straight throughout movement), then reverse the action back to starting position with your back flat on the floor.

(c) Repeat this movement, using your right leg and left hand. Let the abdominal muscles work dynamically and maintain a smooth rhythm throughout.

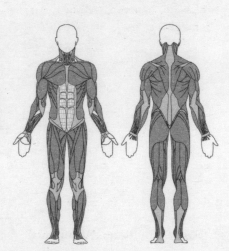

Targets: Abs (Rectus Abdominis)

Cheating V-Ups

The Cheating V-Up is used to develop muscular strength and endurance of the core. Emphasis is placed on the Abs.

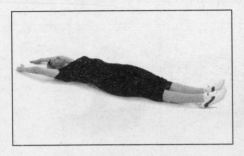 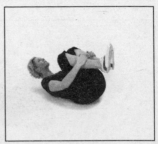

INSTRUCTIONS

(a) Start by lying on your back (supine), with your arms out straight above your head.

(b) Simultaneously raise your legs and torso until you can clasp your knees with your hands in a 'hug' position. Reverse this action back to the starting position to complete one repetition. This exercise is performed in a smooth, controlled action.

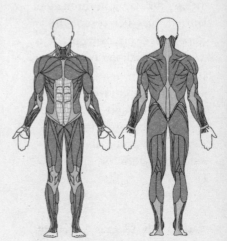

Targets: Abs (Rectus Abdominis)

Plank

The Plank is used to develop muscular strength and endurance of the core. Emphasis is placed on the Abs as they statically contract to maintain integrity in the hold.

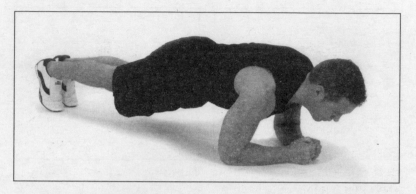

INSTRUCTIONS

(a) Rise onto the balls of your feet held a hip-width apart and stabilise your upper body with the elbows positioned below your shoulders, fingers clasped. Maintain a straight line from head to heel. Contract your abdominals to prevent sagging in the midsection or the opposite with your backside sticking up.

(b) This position will be held statically for a designated time period, usually 30-90 seconds. It is important to maintain proper form throughout, focusing on engaging your abdominals and not compromising form in any way.

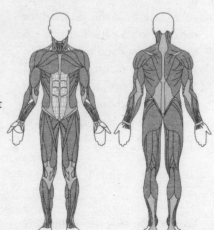

Targets: Abs (Rectus Abdominis)

Plank Plus Raised Leg

This progression of the Plank (above) is used to develop muscular strength and endurance of the core. Emphasis is placed on the Abs as they statically contract to maintain integrity in the hold.

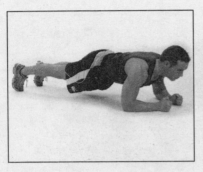 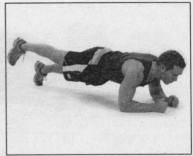

INSTRUCTIONS

(a) With your feet a hip-width apart, rise onto the balls and stabilise your upper body with your elbows positioned below your shoulders, hands clasped. Maintain a straight line from head to heel. Contract your abdominals to prevent sagging in the midsection and avoid the backside sticking up.

(b) Raise one leg until in line with your body, hold this position for the designated period of time and then swap legs and repeat. It is important to maintain proper form throughout, focusing on engaging the abdominals and not compromising form in any way.

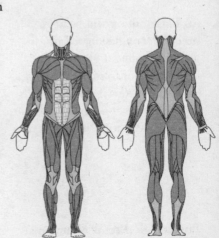

Targets: Abs (Rectus Abdominis)

Side Plank

The Side Plank is used to develop muscular strength and endurance of the core. Emphasis is placed on the Side Abs (Obliques) as they statically contract to maintain integrity in the hold.

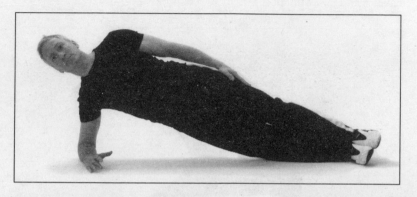

INSTRUCTIONS

(a) Lie on your side, raise the hips and support your upper body with one forearm. The elbow is bent and directly under your shoulder with fingers pointing away. Maintain a straight line from head to toe. Engage the side abs to maintain the integrity of the position and hold for the designated time.

(b) Repeat this process with the other forearm for the same amount of time.

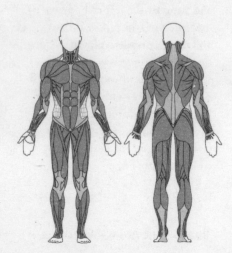

Targets: Side Abs (Obliques)

Side Plank Plus Leg Raise

The Side Plank Plus Leg Raise is used to develop muscular strength and core endurance. This exercise represents a more difficult version to the standard Side Plank (above) and promotes further benefits in balance and co-ordination.

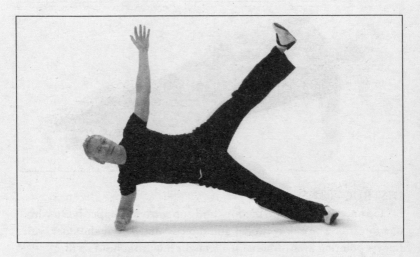

INSTRUCTIONS

(a) Lie on your side, raise your hips and support the upper body with one forearm (the elbow is bent and directly under your shoulder, fingers pointing away). Keep a straight line from head to toe and simultaneously raise the right leg. Engage the abdominals to maintain the integrity of the position. Hold for designated time on both sides.

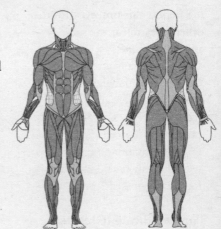

Targets: Side Abs (Obliques)

Side Plank Rotator

The Side Plank Rotator is used to develop muscular strength and endurance of the core. Emphasis is placed on the side abs. This is a more difficult variation on the Side Plank (page 99) as it involves rotation while holding isometrically.

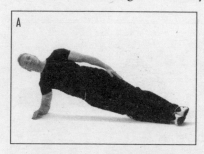

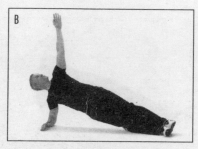

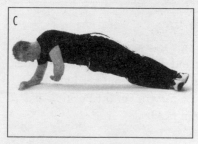

INSTRUCTIONS

(a) Lie on your right side, raise the hips and support your upper body with the right forearm (keep your elbow bent and directly under your shoulder, with fingers pointing away). Maintain a straight line from head to toe.

(b) Straighten your left arm above you.

(c) Now rotate your body and bring the hand to your right hip, sweeping the left arm down (the rest of the body remains fixed in position). Contract the abdominals for two seconds and return to B, with the arm extended. Complete for the designated repetitions.

Targets: Side Abs (Obliques)

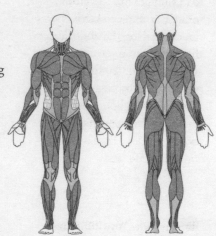

Side Plank Plus Twist

The Side Plank Plus Twist is used to develop muscular strength and endurance of the core. Emphasis is placed on the Side Abs. This is a more difficult variation to the Side Plank (page 99) as it involves rotation while holding isometrically.

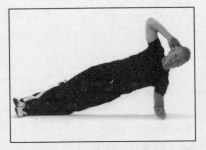
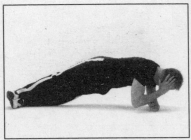

INSTRUCTIONS

(a) Lie on your right side, raise your hips and support the upper body with your forearm (the elbow is bent and directly under your shoulder, with fingers pointing away). Keep a straight line from head to toe. Engage the abdominals to maintain the integrity of the position and place your left palm on the side of your head.

(b) Leading with the elbow, rotate the trunk towards the floor, engaging the abdominals throughout and return to the start position. Complete repetitions, keeping a smooth rhythm throughout and then repeat on the opposite side.

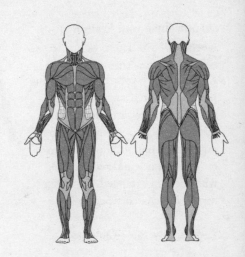

Targets: Side Abs (Obliques)

Side Bridge

The Side Bridge is used to develop muscular strength and endurance of the core. Emphasis is placed on the Side Abs.

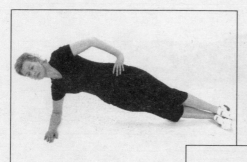

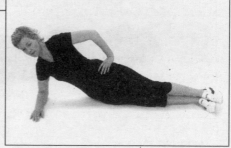

INSTRUCTIONS
(a) Adopt the same position as the side plank (see page 99)

(b) Drop the hips to the floor then contract the side abs to return to start position – this constitutes one repetition. Complete reps for that side then alternate to the other. Maintain a smooth rhythm throughout.

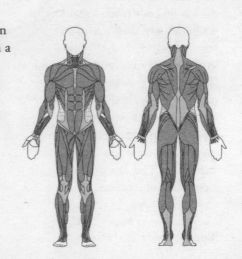

Targets: Side Abs (Obliques)

Dorsal Raise

The Dorsal Raise is used to develop muscular strength and endurance of the core. Emphasis is placed on the lower back.

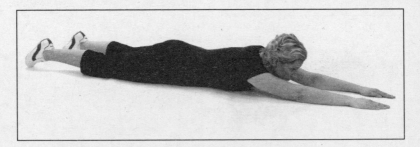

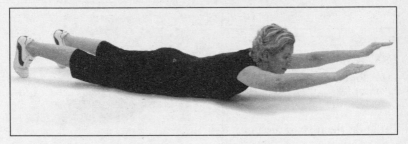

INSTRUCTIONS

(a) Lie on your front, legs straight and arms stretched out in front.

(b) Now lift your head, chest and arms off the ground until you feel your lower back tighten (keep your feet in contact with the floor throughout). Return to start position to complete one repetition. This is a slow and controlled movement.

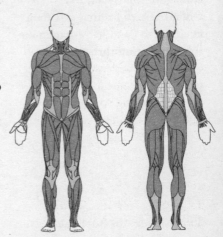

Targets: Lower back (Erector Spinae)

Superman

The Superman is used to develop muscular strength and endurance of the core. Emphasis is placed on the lower back

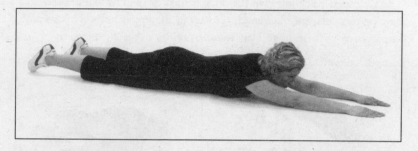

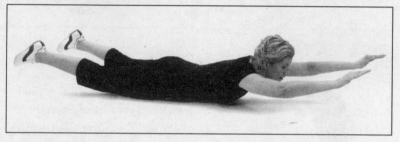

INSTRUCTIONS

(a) Lie on your front, legs straight and arms stretched out in front.

(b) Simultaneously lift your head, chest, arms and legs off the ground to assume a 'Superman' position, feeling your lower back tighten. Return to start position. This is a slow and controlled movement.

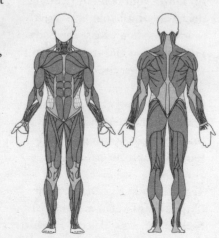

Targets: Lower back (Erector Spinae)

PLYOMETRIC EXERCISES

Extended Kneeling Plyo Press Up

The Extended Kneeling Plyo Press Up is medium intensity and used to develop muscular speed strength (power) in the upper body. This exercise improves co-ordination and the muscles' ability to react explosively.

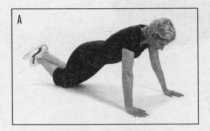

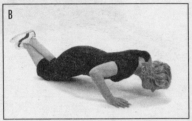

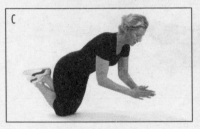

INSTRUCTIONS
(a) Support your body on your knees and cross your feet behind you. Place your hands directly under and shoulder-width apart, maintaining a straight back.

(b) Lower your body by bending the elbows until your chest nearly touches the floor. Keep the body prone without allowing the hips to sag by engaging the core muscles.

(c) As you straighten your elbows on the return, push yourself away from the floor creating enough room to clap your hands.

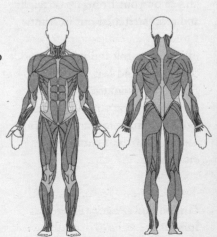

Targets: Chest (Pectorals), front of shoulders (Anterior Deltoids), back of the arms (Triceps Brachii)

Press Up with Hand Clap

The Press Up with Hand Clap is used to develop muscular speed strength (power) in the upper body. This high-intensity exercise improves co-ordination and your muscles' ability to react explosively.

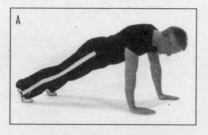

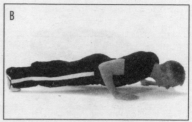

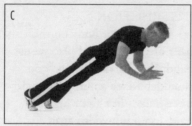

INSTRUCTIONS
(a) Support your body on the balls of your feet and place your hands directly under and shoulder-width apart, your back in a straight line from head to heel, feet a hip-width apart.

(b) Lower your body by bending the elbows until your chest nearly touches the floor. Keep the body prone without allowing the hips to sag by engaging the core muscles.

(c) As you straighten your elbows on the return, push yourself away from the floor creating enough room to clap your hands before returning to the start.

Targets: Chest (Pectorals), front of shoulders (Anterior Deltoids), back of the arms (Triceps Brachii)

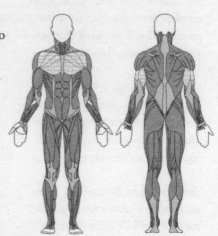

Press Up with Chest Slap

The Press Up with Chest Slap is used to develop muscular speed strength (power) in the upper body. This high-intensity exercise improves co-ordination and the ability of your muscles to react explosively.

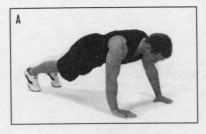

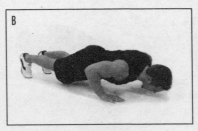

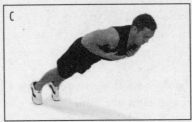

INSTRUCTIONS

(a) Support your body on the balls of your feet and place your hands directly under and shoulder-width apart, your back in a straight line from head to heel, feet a hip-width apart.

(b) Lower your body by bending the elbows until your chest nearly touches the floor. Keep the body prone without allowing the hips to sag by engaging the core muscles.

(c) Straighten your elbows on the return, push yourself forcefully away from the floor creating enough room to slap your chest before returning to the start position.

Targets: Chest (Pectorals), front of shoulders (Anterior Deltoids), back of arms (Triceps Brachii)

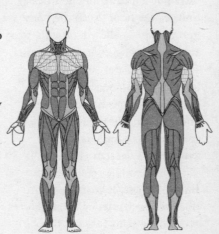

Jumping Jacks

Jumping Jacks are used to develop muscular speed strength (power) in the upper and lower body. They are a low-intensity exercise so ideal for longer intervals or multiple reps. Ideal for all-round fitness and often used as a component of the warm-up.

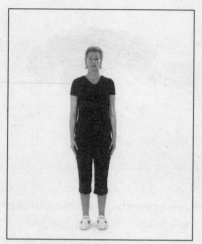 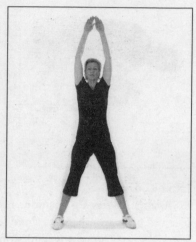

INSTRUCTIONS

(a) Stand with your feet a hip-width apart, keeping a neutral spine (straight back) and with your knees slightly bent and hands by your sides.

(b) Jump and simultaneously raise your hands above your head, spreading your feet laterally by about one-and-a-half shoulder widths. Quickly reverse the movement and repeat.

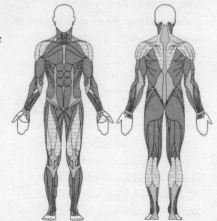

Targets: Shoulders (Deltoids), front of thighs (Quadriceps), upper back (Trapezius), calves (Gastrocnemius)

Mountain Climbers

The Mountain Climber is used to develop muscular speed strength (power) in the lower body. This medium-intensity exercise improves co-ordination and the ability of your muscles to react explosively.

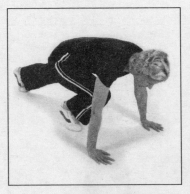

INSTRUCTIONS

(a) Assume a Press Up position: support your body on the balls of your feet and place your hands a shoulder-width apart, keeping your back in a straight line (prone position) from head to toe. Drive one knee up towards your chest.

(b) Quickly jump and exchange legs, keeping a straight back throughout to avoid your backside rising up.

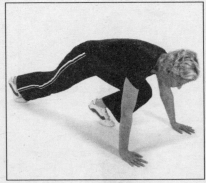

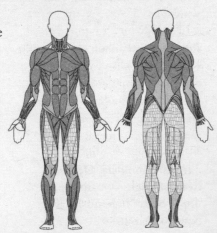

Targets: Front of thighs (Quadriceps), back of thighs (Hamstrings), calves (Gastrocnemius), Glutes (Gluteus Maximus)

Tuck Jumps

The Tuck Jump is used to develop muscular speed strength (power) in the lower body. This high-intensity exercise improves co-ordination and the ability of the muscles to react explosively.

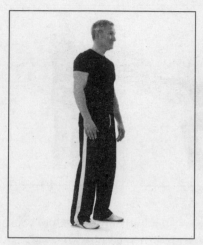

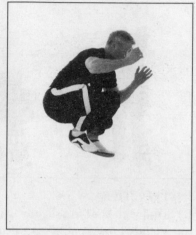

INSTRUCTIONS

(a) Stand with your feet a hip-width apart, keeping a neutral spine (straight back) and with your knees slightly bent and arms in preparation to jump.

(b) Explode into a jump, drawing your knees into your chest and land on the balls of your feet. Repeat for designated repetitions.

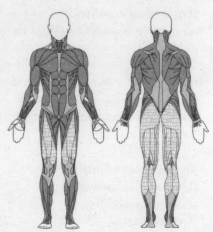

Targets: Front of thighs (Quadriceps), back of thighs (Hamstrings), Calves (Gastrocnemius), Glutes (Gluteus Maximus)

Jump Squats

The Jump Squat is used to develop muscular speed strength (power) in the lower body. This high-intensity exercise improves co-ordination and the ability of your muscles to react explosively.

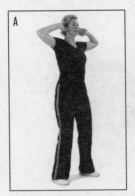
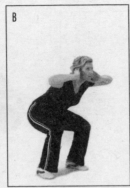
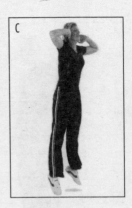

INSTRUCTIONS

(a) Stand with your feet slightly wider than a hip-width apart and the toes slightly turned out. Keep a neutral spine (straight back), knees slightly bent and place your palms behind your head with the elbows elevated (or place hands beside your head).

(b) Now lower yourself under control by bending at the knees until your thighs are parallel to the floor. Push your backside out and contract the abdominals (avoid the knees coming over the toes).

(c) As you rise up, jump vertically in the air (strive to get as high as you can). Land on the balls of your feet and lower yourself into another squat.

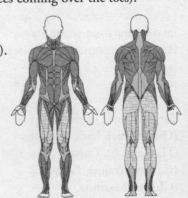

Targets: Front of thighs (Quadriceps), back of thighs (Hamstrings), Calves (Gastrocnemius), Glutes

Squat Kicks

Squat Kicks are used to develop muscular speed strength (power) in the lower body. This medium-intensity exercise improves co-ordination and the ability of your muscles to react explosively.

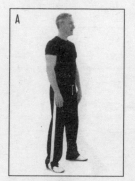
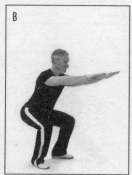
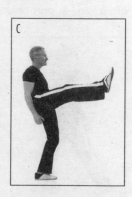

INSTRUCTIONS

(a) Stand with your feet somewhat wider than hip-width apart, with toes slightly turned out. Keep a neutral spine, knees slightly bent and arms extended ahead at shoulder level to stabilise you.

(b) Lower yourself under control by bending the knees until your thighs are parallel with floor. Push your backside out and contract the abdominals, avoid the knees coming over the toes. As with a regular full squat you extend at the knees to return to your starting position,

(c) In this instance as you approach your original position execute a forward kick (raise your thigh and flick your lower leg by again extending the knee). Squat and repeat with opp[osite leg.

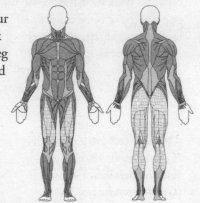

Targets: Front of thighs (Quadriceps), back of thighs (Hamstrings), Calves (Gastrocnemius), Glutes (Gluteus Maximus)

Split Jumps

Split Jumps are used to develop muscular speed strength (power) in the lower body and are considered a low-intensity plyometric exercise ideal for longer intervals or multiple reps. Perfect for all-round fitness and often used as part of the warm-up.

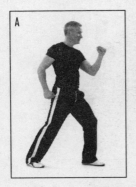
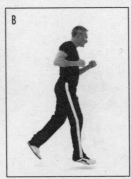
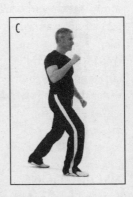

INSTRUCTIONS

(a) Stand with your feet in a 'split' position with one leg forward, the other back, both knees bent. Arms bent at 90 degrees.

(b) Rapidly switch feet by jumping and exchanging positions while driving with the arms.

(c) Land with your feet in the opposite position. This action results in a fast cross-country skiing type action.

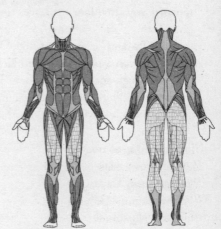

Targets: Front of thighs (Quadriceps), back of thighs (Hamstrings), Calves (Gastrocnemius), Glutes (Gluteus Maximus)

High Knees

High Knees are used to develop muscular speed strength (power) in the lower body and are considered a low-intensity plyometric exercise ideal for longer intervals or multiple reps. Perfect for all-round fitness and often used as part of the warm-up.

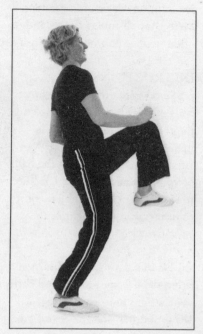

INSTRUCTIONS

(a) Stand with your feet slightly wider than a hip-width apart, with the toes facing forward and maintain a neutral spine (straight back). Rise onto the balls of the feet and lift your left knee towards your chest, simultaneously transferring your weight onto your right leg.

(b) Rapidly bring your left knee down and shift your weight to the left leg, while raising the right knee. This action involves hopping from one foot to the other, lifting your knees high in the process. The end product is a dynamic movement.

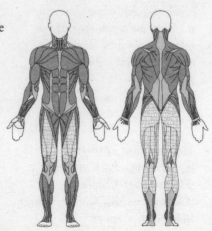

Targets: Front of thighs (Quadriceps), back of thighs (Hamstrings), Calves (Gastrocnemius), Glutes (Gluteus Maximus)

High Knees Plus Skip

High Knees are used to develop muscular speed strength (power) in the lower body. This low-intensity plyometric variation is ideal for longer intervals or multiple reps. Perfect for all-round fitness and often used as part of the warm-up.

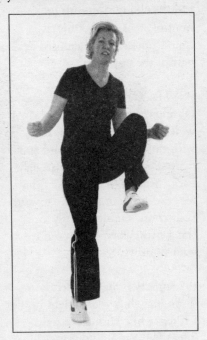

INSTRUCTIONS

(a) Stand with your feet slightly wider than a hip-width apart and the toes facing forward, while maintaining a neutral spine (straight back). Rise onto the balls of your feet and lift your left knee towards your chest simultaneously transferring your weight onto your right leg.

(b) Now make a small skip, then bring the left knee down and shift your weight onto the left leg. Make another small skip and raise your right knee. This action involves quickly hopping and skipping from one foot to the other, lifting your knees high in the process. Like the previous exercise, the end product is a dynamic movement.

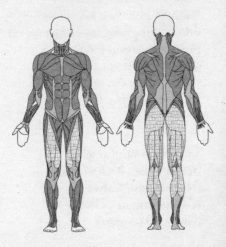

Targets: Front of thighs (Quadriceps), Back of thighs (Hamstrings), Calves (Gastrocnemius), Glutes (Gluteus Maximus)

Lunge Jumps

The Lunge Jump is used to develop muscular speed strength (power) in the lower body. This high-intensity exercise improves co-ordination and the ability of your muscles to react explosively.

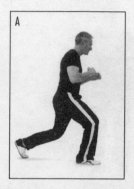
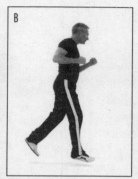
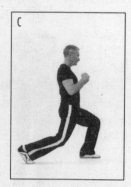

INSTRUCTIONS

(a) Take a long comfortable stride forward (about 91cm/3ft). Now bend the knee and lower yourself towards the floor, keeping the body straight and maintaining a neutral spine (straight back) with your elbows bent at 90 degrees. Ensure your knee does not come over your toe.

(b) Explode into a jump straight up while thrusting your arms forward (keep the elbows bent). Mid-air, switch legs in a scissor action to land in the opposite lunge position. Continue by jumping and switching legs to complete repetitions. The lunge phase should be smooth and controlled, the jump phase explosive.

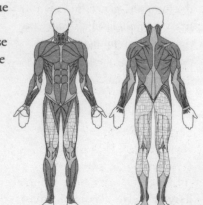

Targets: Front of thighs (Quadriceps), back of thighs (Hamstrings), Calves (Gastrocnemius), Glutes (Gluteus Maximus)

Ankle Jumps

The low-intensity Ankle Jump is used to develop muscular speed strength (power) in the lower body.

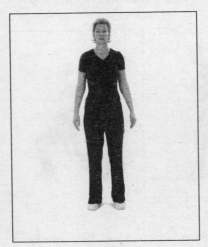 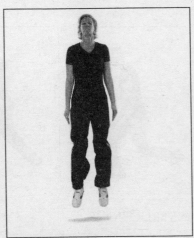

INSTRUCTIONS

(a) Stand with your feet a shoulder-width apart, keeping a neutral spine (straight back) and with your knees slightly bent and hands by your sides.

(b) Jump up, generating the force from your ankles. Pull your core tight while jumping and land on the balls of your feet. Repeat.

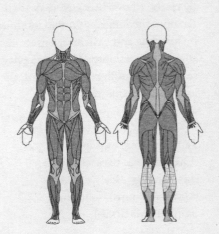

Targets: Calves (Gastrocnemius)

Alternate Toe-Taps

Alternate Toe-Taps are used to develop muscular speed strength (power) in the upper body. They are considered a low-intensity exercise ideal for longer intervals or multiple reps. Perfect for all-round fitness and often used as part of the warm-up.

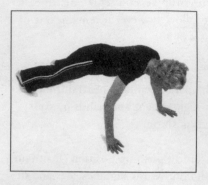 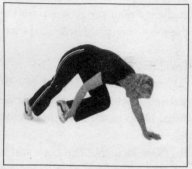

INSTRUCTIONS

(a) Support your body on the balls of the feet and place your hands directly under and a shoulder-width apart. Keep your back in a straight line (prone position) from head to toe.

(b) From this position, simultaneously bring the right hand to the left foot, then immediately alternate with left hand to right foot. The movement should be executed with speed while not compromising form.

Targets: Chest (Pectorals), front of shoulders (Anterior Deltoids), back of the arms (Triceps Brachii), Abs (Rectus Abdominis)

Standard Burpee

The Burpee is one of the most challenging bodyweight exercises you can perform. It incorporates so many major muscle groups while taxing your aerobic and anaerobic systems. This high-intensity movement develops strength, endurance, balance, co-ordination and explosive power. The standard non press-up version represents an easier challenge than the progressions that follow, however it remains one of the most singularly beneficial exercises of all.

INSTRUCTIONS

(a) Stand with your feet a hip-width apart, keeping a neutral spine (straight back) and with your knees slightly bent and hands by your sides. Drop to the floor into a crouch position.

(b) Now kick your legs back and assume a press-up position (maintain a straight line from head to toe, with your hands slightly wider and in line with your shoulders).

(c) Immediately return your feet to the crouch position while simultaneously pushing with the arms. Now jump as high as possible generating force from your legs and extending your arms overhead to land on the balls of your feet.

Targets: Chest (Pectorals), front of shoulders (Anterior Deltoids), back of the arms (Triceps Brachii), Abs (Rectus Abdominis), front of thighs (Quadriceps), Glutes (Gluteus Maximus), back of legs (Hamstrings), Calves (Gastrocnemius)

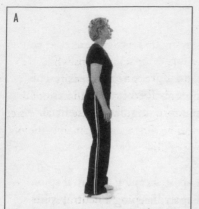

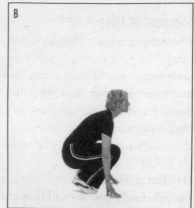

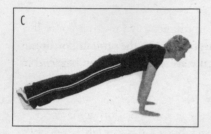

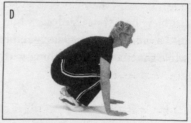

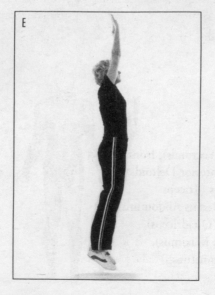

The Burpee (Non-Jump)
Plyometric exercise (High Intensity)

The non-jump version of the Standard Burpee (above) represents an easier challenge than the other progressions featured in this book, however it remains one of the most singularly beneficial bodyweight exercises.

INSTRUCTIONS
(a) Stand with your feet a hip-width apart, keeping a neutral spine (straight back) and with the knees slightly bent and hands by your sides. Drop to the floor in a crouch position

(b) Now kick your legs back while simultaneously lowering yourself into a press-up. Immediately return your feet to the crouch position, while simultaneously pushing with the arms. Finish as you began.

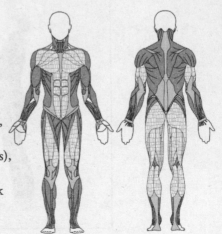

Targets: Chest (Pectorals), front of shoulders (Anterior Deltoids), back of the arms (Triceps Brachii), Abs (Rectus Abdominis), front of thighs (Quadriceps), Glutes (Gluteus Maximus), back of the legs (Hamstrings), Calves (Gastrocnemius)

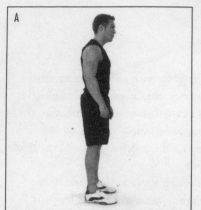

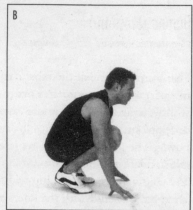

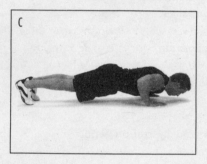

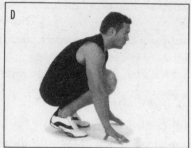

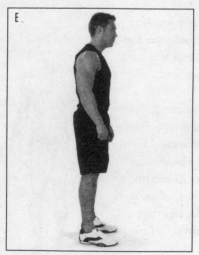

Burpee (Press Up)
Plyometric exercise (High Intensity)

The Burpee is one of the most challenging bodyweight exercises you can perform. It incorporates many major muscle groups of the body whilst taxing both your aerobic and anaerobic systems. This movement develops strength, endurance, balance, co-ordination and explosive power. The press up version represents a more difficult challenge than the standard and non-jump variations.

INSTRUCTIONS
(a) Stand with your feet hip width apart, keeping a neutral spine, knees slightly bent and hands by your sides.

(b) Drop to the floor into a crouch position

(c) Kick your legs back while simultaneously lowering yourself into a press-up

(d) Immediately return your feet to crouch position, while simultaneously pushing with the arms.

(e) Jump as high as possible generating force from your legs extend arms overhead and land on the balls of your feet.

Targets: Chest (Pectorals), Front of shoulders (Anterior Deltoids), Back of arms (Triceps Brachii), Abs (Rectus Abdominis), Front of thighs (Quadriceps) Glutes (Gluteus Maximus), Back of legs (Hamstrings), Calves (Gastrocnemius)

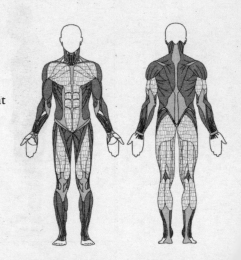

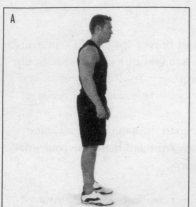

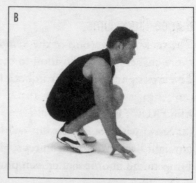

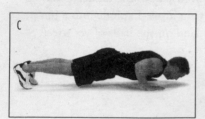

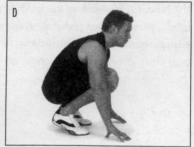

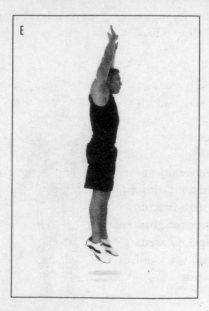

Burpee (Tuck Jump)

The tuck jump version of the Standard Burpee (page 120) represents a more challenging proposition to the standard Burpee and specifically develops significant power in both legs.

INSTRUCTIONS

(a) Stand with your feet a hip-width apart, keeping a neutral spine (straight back) with your knees slightly bent and hands by your sides. Drop to the floor into a crouch position.

(b) Now kick your legs back while simultaneously lowering yourself into a press up. Immediately return your feet to the crouch position, while simultaneously pushing with your arms. Explode into a jump, pull your knees into your chest and land on the balls of your feet.

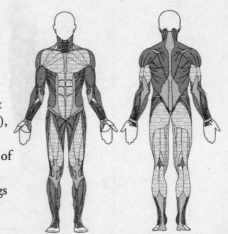

Targets: Chest (Pectorals), front of shoulders (Anterior Deltoids), back of arms (Triceps Brachii), Abs (Rectus Abdominis), front of thighs (Quadriceps), Glutes (Gluteus Maximus), back of legs (Hamstrings), Calves (Gastrocnemius)

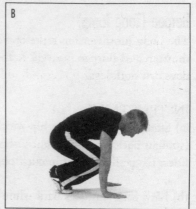

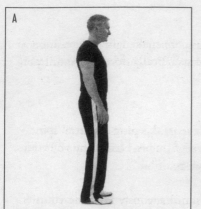

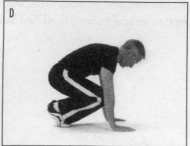

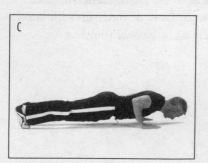

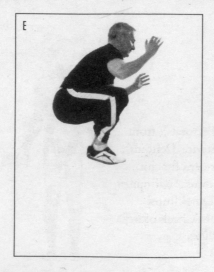

Burpee (Long Jump)

The Long Jump version represents a more challenging proposition to the Standard Burpee (page 120) and specifically develops significant power in both legs.

INSTRUCTIONS

(a) Stand with your feet a hip-width apart, keeping a neutral spine (straight back) and with your knees slightly bent and hands by your sides. Drop to the floor into a crouch position.

(b) Kick your legs back while simultaneously lowering yourself into a press up. Immediately return your feet to the crouch position while simultaneously pushing with your arms. Explode into a forward jump, extend your arms overhead and land on the balls of your feet.

Targets: Chest (Pectorals), front of shoulders (Anterior Deltoids), back of the arms (Triceps Brachii), Abs (Rectus Abdominis), front of thighs (Quadriceps), Glutes (Gluteus Maximus), back of legs (Hamstrings), Calves (Gastrocnemius)

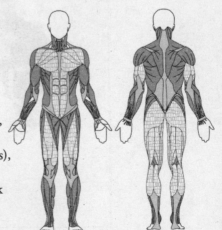

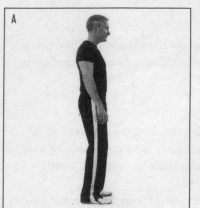

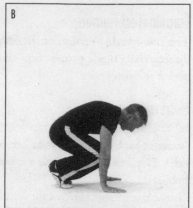

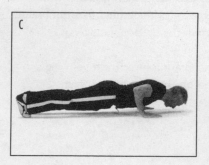

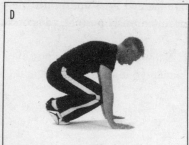

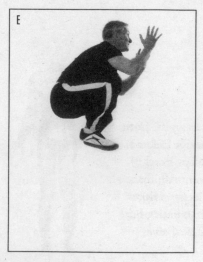

One-Handed Burpee

The one-handed version of the Standard Burpee (page 120) represents a more challenging proposition and specifically develops significant power in either arm.

INSTRUCTIONS

(a) Stand with your feet a hip-width apart, keeping a neutral spine (straight back) and with your knees slightly bent and hands by your sides. Drop to the floor into a crouch position, supporting with one hand.

(b) Kick your legs back while simultaneously lowering yourself into a one-handed press up. Immediately return to the crouch position, while simultaneously pushing with one arm.

(c) Now jump as high as possible, generating force from your legs. Extend your arms overhead and land on the balls of your feet.

Targets: Chest (Pectorals), front of shoulders (Anterior Deltoids), back of arms (Triceps Brachii), Abs (Rectus Abdominis), front of thighs (Quadriceps), Glutes (Gluteus Maximus), back of the legs (Hamstrings), Calves (Gastrocnemius)

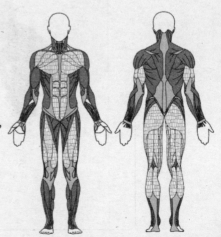

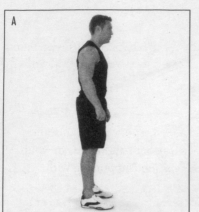

A

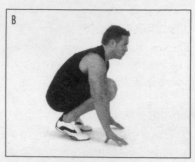

B

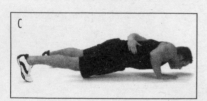

C

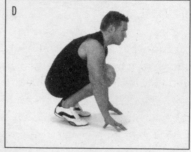

D

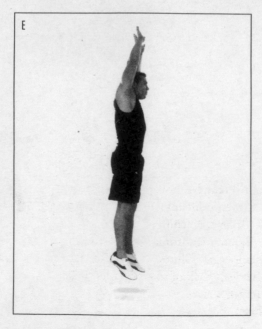

E

Chapter Five

LEVEL 1

Important Note: Level 1 is intended for those who have built a base level of fitness and who are accustomed to some recent exercise.

If you are completely new to exercise, unfit or leading a sedentary lifestyle, please re-read the Introduction to Physical Fitness (Chapter Two) and take initial steps towards building a platform of fitness. The workouts in *5 Minute Fitness* are demanding and will involve your heart, lungs and muscles working at a high intensity: it is for this reason that a certain level of conditioning is required before moving forward. Even for those who have a base level of fitness, working at maximal- or near-maximal intensity will be uncharted territory, so I will gradually introduce you to intensity in Level 1 in preparation for the next two levels.

GPP workouts (see also page 3) are challenging and will involve a high output of energy, not maximal- but high-intensity, whereas HIIT Tabata intervals are by nature ultra-intense and involve working at complete maximal intensity. In this level, we will introduce Tabata but not in its complete form: instead of the usual eight-work intervals, I will start you off with two to four in preparation for Level 2. I suggest you use these workouts for six to eight weeks before stepping up to the next level.

These workouts can be used to supplement your existing programme or maintain and even improve your fitness when away or at home. The benefits are consistent throughout and designed to improve your all-round physical fitness (see also pages 7 and 8).

A number of workouts will refer to intensity in the form of Rate of Perceived Exertion (RPE). This method of measuring intensity requires you to self-assess how hard you are working in relation to a numbering system, as listed on page 135. For further information on intensity and how it impacts on your fitness goals, refer to Chapter Two.

You will need a sports timer/stopwatch to complete the timed workouts (the majority of mobile phones have a stopwatch). For Tabata intervals you can download Tabata timers from the Internet (search 'Tabata timer' – there are several to choose from if you search in Google).

Ensure you are wearing appropriate, comfortable sports clothing and footwear to exercise in. Do not exercise immediately after eating: allow at least an hour to digest (two hours is ideal and recommended) before. Ensure you have water available.

Where to Exercise
These workouts have been designed to be performed anywhere, from your living space to hotel room – just ensure the exercise area is free of obstructions and safe to use. Check ceiling height for any jumping that may be involved.

Frequency and Choice of Mini-Workout
If you are using these workouts to supplement your current exercise programme or simply using them occasionally you can select any mini-workout arbitrarily. If you intended to use them as a routine you can do the following: perform one mini-workout per day. Separate GPP (General Physical Preparedness, see also page 3) and bodyweight circuits one day apart and do no more than one Tabata mini-workout per week. You can add a core mini-workout to any day in addition

to your selected workout – perform this immediately afterwards or at a different time during the day. It is important also to give your body a rest so after every 4–6 weeks have a rest week then return to your routine.

Example: Five-day week

Monday	Tuesday	Wednesday	Thursday	Friday
Bodyweight Circuit Core mini-workout	GPP	Tabata Core mini-workout	Bodyweight Circuit	GPP Core mini-workout

Borg CR10 Scale

0	Nothing at all
0.5	Extremely weak (just noticeable)
1	Very weak
2	Weak (light)
3	Moderate
4	Somewhat strong
5	Strong (heavy)
6	
7	Very strong
8	
9	
10	Extremely strong
*	Maximal

Feedback on how you feel and how this relates to the scale:
3 Moderate: Easy to perform
4 Somewhat strong: Fairly easy

5 Strong (heavy): Breathing and working a little hard
6 Stronger: Beginning to breathe heavily
7 Very strong: Very challenging, breathing very hard
8 Working and breathing seriously hard
9 Approaching upper limits, working and breathing at near-maximal intensity
10 Extremely strong: Working and breathing at maximal intensity
Maximal: 100% effort

> **Important:** When using RPE, it is important that you distinguish between the effects of physical fatigue and unsafe signs such as shortness of breath or dizziness. Always monitor yourself properly. Levels of intensity will also be referred to in terms of tempo (speed), as in the bodyweight circuits (high, medium or low).

Level 1: Mini-Workouts

> **Warning:** Please study carefully the information provided at the beginning of this level. If you are new to this kind of rigorous training, take the necessary steps to prepare yourself before starting out. Avoid high-intensity and high-impact exercise if you have any underlying issues with your health or joint problems that may exacerbate your condition.

GPP Workouts (Timed)
Mini-Workout GPP 1
To start: Warm-up (see Chapter Three for a detailed description)
Requires: Timer/stopwatch
For all the workouts in this chapter, refer to Index of Exercises (Chapter Four) for instructions on how to perform specific exercises.

Exercise	Sets	Work (seconds)	Rest (seconds)	Total Time (minutes)
Jumping Jacks	1	30	30	
Standard Squats	1	30	30	
Mountain Climbers	1	30	30	
Extended Kneeling Press Ups	1	30	30	8

Complete two circuits
To finish: Cool down (refer to Chapter Three for a detailed description.

Workout Guide

Start with a warm-up. Perform Jumping Jacks for thirty seconds non-stop at a high intensity (Level 7–8 RPE chart). On completion, rest for thirty seconds then move on to Standard Squats, Mountain Climbers and Kneeling Press Ups (use a variation you can perform for high reps), taking rests of thirty seconds between each exercise. The completion of all four exercises constitutes one circuit. Proceed by completing a further circuit. Cool down gradually and finish with some maintenance and/or developmental stretches.

Progressions

Increase the work time
Increase the circuits
Decrease the rest time.

Mini-Workout GPP 2

To start: Warm-up (see Chapter Three for a detailed description)
Requires: Timer/stopwatch

Exercise	Sets	Work (seconds)	Rest (seconds)	Total Time (minutes)
Standard Squats	1	30	30	
Split Jumps	1	30	30	
Alternate Toe Taps	1	30	30	
Seated Row Crunches	1	30	30	8

Complete two circuits.

To finish: Cool down (refer to Chapter Three for a detailed description.

Workout Guide

Start with a warm-up. Perform squats for thirty seconds non-stop at a high intensity (7–8 on the RPE chart). On completion, take a rest for thirty seconds then move onto Split Jumps, Alternate Toe Taps and Seated Row Crunches. The completion of all four exercises constitutes one circuit. Proceed by completing a further circuit. Cool down gradually and finish with some maintenance and/or developmental stretches.

Progressions

Increase the work time

Increase the circuits

Decrease the rest time.

Mini-Workout GPP 3

To start: Warm-up (see Chapter Three for a detailed description)

Requires: Timer/stopwatch

Exercise	Sets	Work (seconds)	Rest (seconds)	Total Time (minutes)
High Knees	1	30	30	
Standard Squats	1	30	30	
Jumping Jacks	1	30	30	
Cheating V-Ups	1	30	30	8

Complete two circuits.
To finish: Cool down (refer to Chapter Three for a detailed description.

Workout Guide
Start with a warm-up. Perform High Knees for thirty seconds non-stop at a high intensity (7–8 on the RPE chart). On completion, take a rest for 30 seconds then move on to Squats, Jumping Jacks and Cheating V-Ups. The completion of all four exercises constitutes one circuit. Proceed by completing a further circuit. Cool down gradually and finish with some maintenance and/or developmental stretches.

Progressions
Increase the work time
Increase the circuits
Decrease the rest time

Bodyweight Circuits (Reps)

Mini-Workout Bodyweight Circuit 1
To start: Warm-up (see Chapter Three for a detailed description)
Requires: Timer/stopwatch

Exercise	Reps	Tempo	Rest (seconds)
High Knees	60	High	
Squats	15–20	Medium	
Extended Kneeling Press Ups	10–15	Medium	
Crunches	20	Medium	45

Complete two to three circuits.
To finish: Cool down (refer to Chapter Three for a detailed description.

Workout Guide

Start with a warm-up. Perform High Knees for sixty reps non-stop at a high tempo. On completion, move immediately onto squats for fifteen to twenty reps medium tempo, Extended Kneeling Press Ups (or an alternative variation) for ten to fifteen reps medium tempo and end with crunches for twenty reps, medium tempo. All four exercises are performed consecutively without stopping. After one full circuit, rest for forty-five seconds and complete two to three circuits in total. Cool down gradually and finish with some maintenance and/or developmental stretches.

Progressions

Increase the repetitions
Increase the circuits
Decrease the rest period
Select a more challenging variation of exercise than prescribed

Mini-Workout Bodyweight Circuit 2

To start: Warm-up (see Chapter Three for a detailed description)
Requires: Timer/stopwatch

Exercise	Reps	Tempo	Rest (seconds)
Jumping Jacks	50	High	
Prisoner Squats	15–20	Medium	
Extended Kneeling Press Ups	20	Medium	
Floor Bridge	15–20	Medium	45

Complete two to three circuits.
To finish: Cool down (refer to Chapter Three for a detailed description.

Workout Guide

Start with a warm-up. Perform Jumping Jacks for fifty reps non-stop at a high tempo. On completion, move immediately onto Prisoner Squats for fifteen to twenty reps medium tempo, Extended Kneeling Press Ups (or an alternative variation) for twenty reps at a medium tempo and end with the Floor Bridge for fifteen to twenty reps medium tempo. All four exercises are performed consecutively without stopping. After one full circuit, rest for forty-five seconds and complete two to three circuits in total. Cool down gradually and finish with some maintenance and/or developmental stretches.

Progressions
Increase the repetitions
Increase the circuits
Decrease the rest period
Select a more challenging variation of exercise than prescribed

Mini-Workout Bodyweight Circuit 3
To start: Warm-up (see Chapter Three for a detailed description)
Requires: Timer/stopwatch

Exercise	Reps	Tempo	Rest (seconds)
Lunges	20	Medium	
Dolphin Press Ups	10–15	Medium	
Calf Raises	20	Medium	
Bicycle Crunches	20–30	Medium	45

Complete two to three circuits.
To finish: Cool down (refer to Chapter Three for a detailed description.

Workout Guide
Start with a warm-up, then lunges for twenty reps (ten per leg), medium tempo. On completion, move immediately onto Dolphin Press Ups for ten to fifteen reps medium tempo, Calf Raises for twenty reps medium tempo and end with Bicycle Crunches for twenty to thirty reps medium tempo. All four exercises are performed consecutively without stopping. After one full circuit, rest for forty-five seconds and complete two to three circuits in total. Cool down gradually and finish with some maintenance and/or developmental stretches.

Progressions
Increase the repetitions
Increase the circuits
Decrease the rest period
Select a more challenging variation of exercise than prescribed.

Mini-Workout Bodyweight Circuit 4
To start: Warm-up (see Chapter Three for a detailed description)
Requires: Timer/stopwatch

Exercise	Reps	Tempo	Rest (seconds)
Side-to-Side Squat	20	Medium	
Extended Kneeling Press Up	15–20	Medium	
Calf Raises	20–30	High	
Floor Bridge	12–15	Medium	45

Complete two to three circuits.
To finish: Cool down (refer to Chapter Three for a detailed description.

Workout Guide
Start with a warm-up then begin with Side-to-Side Squats for twenty reps (ten per leg) medium tempo. On completion, move immediately onto Extended Kneeling Press Ups for fifteen to twenty reps medium tempo, Calf Raises for twenty to thirty reps medium tempo and end with the Floor Bridge for twelve to fifteen reps medium tempo. All four exercises are performed consecutively without stopping. After one full circuit, rest for forty-five to sixty seconds. Complete two to three circuits in total. Cool down gradually and finish with some maintenance and/or developmental stretches.

Progressions
Increase the repetitions
Increase the circuits
Decrease the rest period
Select a more challenging variation of exercise than prescribed

Mini-Workout Bodyweight Circuit 5

To start: Warm-up (see Chapter Three for a detailed description)

Requires: Timer/stopwatch

Exercise	Reps	Tempo	Rest (seconds)
Wide Squat	15–20	Medium	
Floor Extended Dip	15–20	Medium	
One Leg-Deadlift	10	Medium	
Seated Row Crunch	15–20	Medium	45

Complete two to three circuits.

To finish: Cool down (refer to Chapter Three for a detailed description).

Workout Guide

Start with a warm-up. Begin with Wide Squats for fifteen to twenty reps medium tempo. On completion, move immediately onto Extended Floor Dips for fifteen to twenty reps medium tempo, one Leg Dead-lifts for ten reps (five per leg) medium tempo and end with Seated Row Crunches for fifteen to twenty reps medium tempo. All four exercises are performed consecutively without stopping. After one full circuit, rest for forty-five seconds. Complete two to three circuits in total. Cool down gradually and finish with some maintenance and/or developmental stretches.

Progressions

Increase the repetitions

Increase the circuits

Decrease the rest period

Select a more challenging variation of exercise than prescribed

Introduction to Tabata

Important: Please study the notes on Tabata in Chapter One. The intended protocol is to approach these intervals at maximal intensity for eight cycles. As you will be attempting these mini-workouts for the first time, it is advisable to start off with fewer intervals and work your way up to Tabata Level 2. Strive to exercise at near maximal until you feel comfortable enough to push yourself a little harder.

Mini-Workout: Tabata 1 (Introduction)
To start: Warm-up (see Chapter Three for a detailed description).
Requires: Timer/stopwatch

Exercise	Sets	Interval (seconds)	Rest (seconds)	Minutes
Jumping Jacks	2–4	20	10	
Total time				1–2

To finish: Cool down (refer to Chapter Three for a detailed description).

Workout Guide
Start with a warm-up. Perform Jumping Jacks for twenty seconds at maximal intensity (Level 10 on the RPE chart). Rest for 10 seconds. Now attempt another twenty-second maximal intensity interval: attempt a few more sets if you feel comfortable. Cool down gradually and finish with some maintenance and/or developmental stretches.

Progression
Move up to Level 2 Tabata mini-workouts

Mini-Workout: Muscular Strength and Endurance 'Ladder'
To start: Warm-up (see Chapter Three for a detailed description)
Requires: Timer/stopwatch

Exercise	Reps	Count	Rest (seconds)
Kneeling Press Up	1	1	
	2	2	
	3	3	
	4	4	
	5	5	
			30

Complete two to three circuits.
To finish: Re-warm (refer to Chapter Three for a detailed description).

Workout Guide
Start off with a warm-up. Now begin with a Kneeling Press Up (if this doesn't present enough of a challenge, attempt an Extended Kneeling Press Up* variation). Start by performing one press up, hold in the 'up' position and count for one. Perform two press ups and count for two in the 'up' position. Continue until you reach five reps, followed by a five count. Rest thirty seconds and complete two to three circuits in total. Re-warm gradually and finish with some maintenance and/or developmental stretches.

Progressions
Increase the repetitions
Increase the circuits
Decrease the rest period
Select a more challenging variation of exercise than prescribed

Mini-Workout: Muscular Strength and Endurance 'Ladder'
To start: Warm-up (see Chapter Three for a detailed description)
Requires: Timer/stopwatch

Exercise	Reps	Count	Rest (seconds)
Floor Dip	1	1	
	2	2	
	3	3	
	4	4	
	5	5	
			30

Complete two to three circuits.
To finish: Re-warm (refer to Chapter Three for a detailed description).

Workout Guide
Start with a warm-up, followed by a Floor Dip (if this doesn't present enough of a challenge, attempt a Floor-Extended Dip*/Elevated Dip variation*). Start by performing one Dip, hold in the 'up' position and count for one. Perform two Dips and count two in the 'up' position. Continue until you reach five reps, followed by a five count. Rest for 30 seconds and complete two to three circuits in total. Re-warm gradually (refer to Chapter Three for a detailed description) and finish with some maintenance and/or developmental stretches.

Progressions
Increase the repetitions
Increase the circuits
Decrease the rest period
Select a more challenging variation of exercise than prescribed

Mini-Workout: Plyometric Power-Up Sets

Important: This Plyometric mini-workout is designed to familiarise you with the demands that this form of training places on the body: attempt with caution.

To start: Warm-up (see Chapter Three for a detailed description)
Requires: Timer/stopwatch

Exercise	Sets	Reps	Tempo	Rest (seconds)
Extended Kneeling Plyo Press Ups	2	8–10	High/Explosive	45
Squat Jumps	2	8–10	High/Explosive	45
Ankle Jumps	2	15–20	High/Explosive	45

To finish: Cool down (refer to Chapter Three for a detailed description).

Workout Guide
Start with a warm-up, followed by two sets of Extended Kneeling Plyo Press Ups for eight to ten reps per set (high tempo). Rest for forty-five seconds before completing the second set. Continue with two sets of prescribed Squat Jumps and two sets of prescribed Ankle Jumps, resting forty-five seconds between each set. Cool down gradually and finish with some maintenance and/or developmental stretches.

Progressions
Increase the repetitions
Increase the sets
Decrease the rest period
More challenging plyometric variations appear to Levels 2 and 3 to follow.

Core Workouts
Core Workout 1
To start: Warm-up (see Chapter Three for a detailed description)
Requires: Timer/stopwatch

Exercise	Reps	Rest (seconds)
Abdominal Crunches	20	
Seated Row Crunches	10	
Side Plank	20-second count	
Dorsal Raises	10	30

Repeat circuit three to five times.
To finish: Re-warm (refer to Chapter Three for a detailed description).

Workout Guide

Start with a warm-up. Perform the exercises medium tempo without resting. First, twenty Abdominal Crunches followed by ten Seated Row Crunches and then Side Plank for two x ten-second counts per side, ending with ten Dorsal Raises. Rest for thirty seconds and repeat the circuit three to five times. Re-warm and finish with some maintenance and/or developmental stretches.

Progressions

Increase the repetitions
Increase the circuits
Decrease the rest period
Select a more challenging variation of exercise than prescribed.

Core Workout 2

To start: Warm-up (see Chapter Three for a detailed description)
Requires: Timer/stopwatch

Exercise	Reps	Rest (seconds)
Abdominal Crunches	20	
Russian Twists	20	
Side Bridge	10	
Dorsal Raises	10	30

Repeat circuit three to five times.
To finish: Re-warm (refer to Chapter Three for a detailed description).

Workout Guide
Start with a warm-up. Perform all the exercises medium tempo without resting: twenty Abdominal Crunches followed by twenty Russian Twists, then ten Side Bridges (five reps per side), ending with ten Dorsal Raises. Rest for 30 seconds and then repeat the circuit three to five times. Re-warm and finish with some maintenance and/or developmental stretches.

Progressions
Increase the repetitions
Increase the circuits
Decrease the rest period
Select a more challenging variation of exercise than prescribed.

Core Workout 3
To start: Warm-up (see Chapter Three for a detailed description)
Requires: Timer/stopwatch

Exercise	Reps	Rest (seconds)
Cheating V-Ups	10	
Reverse Crunches	10	
Oblique Seated Row Crunch	20	
Bicycle Crunches	20	30

Repeat circuit three to five times.
To finish: Re-warm (refer to Chapter Three for a detailed description).

Workout Guide
Start off with a warm-up. Perform all the exercises medium tempo without resting: ten Cheating V-Ups followed by ten Reverse Crunches and then twenty Oblique Seated Row Crunches (ten per side), finishing with 20 Bicycle Crunches. Rest for thirty seconds and repeat the circuit three to five times. Re-warm and finish with some maintenance and/or developmental stretches.

Progressions

Increase the repetitions

Increase the circuits

Decrease the rest period

Select a more challenging variation of exercise than prescribed.

Core Workout 4

To start: Warm-up (see Chapter Three for a detailed description)

Requires: Timer/stopwatch

Exercise	Reps	Rest (seconds)
Raised Leg Crunches	20	
Alternate V-Ups	10	
Windscreen Wipers	20	
Superman	10	30

Repeat circuit three to five times.

To finish: Re-warm (refer to Chapter Three for a detailed description)

Workout Guide

Start with a warm-up then perform all the exercises without resting. First, twenty Raised Leg Crunches followed by ten Alternate V-Ups, then twenty Windscreen Wipers (ten per side), finishing with ten Superman. Rest for thirty seconds and repeat the circuit three to five times. Re-warm and finish with some maintenance and/or developmental stretches.

Progressions

Increase the repetitions

Increase the circuits

Decrease the rest period

Select a more challenging variation of exercise than prescribed

Chapter Six

LEVEL 2

Important Note: The workouts in this level pose a significant challenge and include more technically difficult exercises and progressions. The Burpee, for example, will test you aerobically and anaerobically in equal measure, improving muscular strength and endurance but also speed strength (power).

Level 2 is suited to the regular exerciser who might usually go to the gym two to three times per week. If you are new to exercising at a high intensity, you may want to start at Level 1 initially and progress. This level involves more advanced GPP, Bodyweight and Tabata workouts, as well as Little Method workouts (an alternative HIIT regimen using different parameters with similar training benefits).

These workouts can be used to supplement your existing programme or maintain and even improve your fitness away or at home. I suggest that you use the workouts for six to eight weeks before stepping up to the next stage. The benefits of these workouts are consistent throughout and designed to improve your all-round physical fitness (see also pages 7-8 for the benefits of *5 Minute Fitness* workouts).

A number of workouts will refer to intensity in the form of Rate of Perceived Exertion (RPE). This method of measuring intensity requires you to self-assess how hard you are working in relation to the numbering system as listed on page 153. For further information on intensity and how it impacts on your fitness goals, refer to Chapter Two.

You will need a sports timer/stopwatch to complete the timed workouts (the majority of mobile phones have a stopwatch). For Tabata intervals you can download Tabata timers from the Internet (search 'Tabata timer' – there are several to choose from in Google).

Ensure you are wearing appropriate clothing and footwear to exercise in. Do not exercise immediately after eating: allow at least an hour to digest (two hours is ideal and recommended) before. Ensure you have water available.

Where to Exercise

These workouts have been designed to be performed anywhere from your living space to hotel room. Just ensure your exercise area is clear of obstructions and safe to use – check the ceiling height for any jumping that may be involved.

Frequency and Choice of Mini-Workout

Perform one mini-workout per day.

Separate different mini-workouts one day apart and do no more than one Tabata mini-workout per week. You can also add a core mini-workout to any day in addition to your selected workout: perform this immediately afterwards or at a different time during the day.

Example: Five-day week

Monday	Tuesday	Wednesday	Thursday	Friday
Bodyweight Circuit	GPP	Tabata	Bodyweight Circuit	Little Method
Core mini-workout		Core mini-workout		Core mini-workout

Borg CR10 Scale

0	Nothing at all
0.5	Extremely weak (just noticeable)
1	Very weak
2	Weak (light)
3	Moderate
4	Somewhat strong
5	Strong (heavy)
6	
7	Very strong
8	
9	
10	Extremely strong
*	Maximal

Feedback on how you feel and how this relates to the scale:

3 Moderate: Easy to perform

4 Somewhat strong: Fairly easy

5 Strong (heavy): Breathing and working a little hard

6 Stronger: Beginning to breathe heavily

7 Very strong: Very challenging, breathing very hard

8 Working and breathing seriously hard

9 Approaching upper limits, working and breathing at near maximal intensity

10 Extremely strong: Working and breathing at maximal intensity

*Maximal: 100% effort

Important: When using RPE, it is important that you distinguish between the effects of physical fatigue and unsafe signs such as shortness of breath or dizziness. Always monitor yourself properly. Levels of intensity will also be referred to in terms of tempo (speed) as in the bodyweight circuits (high, medium or low).

Level 2: Mini-Workouts

> **Important:** Please study carefully the information provided at the beginning of this level (page 151). If you are new to this kind of rigorous training, take the necessary steps to prepare yourself before starting out. If you have any underlying issues with your health or joint problems, avoid high-intensity and high-impact exercise that may exacerbate your condition

Bodyweight Circuits (Reps)

Bodyweight Circuit 1

To start: Warm-up (see Chapter Three for a detailed description)

Requires: Timer/stopwatch

For all the workouts in this chapter, refer to Index of Exercises (Chapter Four) for instructions on how to perform specific exercises.

Exercise	Reps	Tempo	Rest (seconds)
High Knees	60	High	
Standard Press Ups	15–20	Medium	
Wide Squats	15–20	Medium	
Seated Row Crunches	20	Medium	
Squat Hold	30-second count	Static	
Squat Jumps	8–10	High	30–45

Complete two to three circuits.

To finish: Cool down (refer to Chapter Three for a detailed description).

Workout Guide

Start with a warm-up. All the exercises are performed consecutively without a break. The completion of all six exercises constitutes one circuit, rest thirty to forty-five seconds and repeat for a further one to two circuits. High Knees should be approached at a high tempo for sixty reps, then Standard Press Ups for fifteen to twenty reps (if these prove too easy, select a more difficult variation). Follow with Wide Squats for fifteen to twenty reps at a medium tempo, Seated Row Crunches for twenty reps (medium tempo) and into a Squat Hold for thirty seconds (time or count thirty seconds). End with Squat Jumps for eight to ten reps. Cool down and finish with some maintenance and/or developmental stretches.

Progressions
Increase the repetitions
Increase the circuits
Decrease the rest period.

Bodyweight Circuit 2
To start: Warm-up (see Chapter Three for a detailed description)
Requires: Timer/stopwatch

Exercise	Reps	Tempo	Rest (seconds)
Jumping Jacks	50	High	
Spiderman Press Ups	15–20	Medium	
Cheating V-Ups	20	Medium	
Standard Burpee variation	8–10	High	
Alternate Lunges	20	Medium	
Plank	30–45 second count	Static	30–45

Complete two to three circuits.
To finish: Cool down (refer to Chapter Three for a detailed description).

Workout Guide
Start with a warm-up. All exercises are performed consecutively without a break. The completion of all six exercises constitutes one circuit, rest thirty to forty-five seconds and repeat for a further one to two circuits. Jumping Jacks should be approached at a high tempo for fifty reps, then

Spiderman Press Ups for fifteen to twenty reps, Cheating V-Ups for twenty reps at a medium tempo, Standard Burpee variation for eight to ten reps at a high tempo and into Lunges for twenty reps at a medium tempo. End with a Plank Hold (time or count for thirty to forty-five seconds). Cool down and finish with some maintenance and/or developmental stretches.

Progressions

Increase the repetitions
Increase the circuits
Increase the Plank hold time
Decrease the rest period.

Bodyweight Circuit 3

To start: Warm-up (see Chapter Three for a detailed description)
Requires: Timer/stopwatch

Exercise	Reps	Tempo	Rest (seconds)
Split Jumps	60	High	
Bulgarian Squats	20	Medium	
Hindu Press Ups	10	Medium	
Bicycle Crunches	30	Medium	
Burpee (Non-Jump) variation	8–10	High	
Superman	15	Slow	30–45

Complete two to three circuits
To finish: Cool down

Workout Guide

Start with a warm-up. All exercises are performed consecutively without rest. The completion of all six exercises constitutes one circuit. Rest thirty to forty-five seconds and repeat for a further one to two circuits. Split Jumps should be approached at a high tempo for sixty reps, then Bulgarian Squats for twenty reps (ten per lag) at a medium tempo. Follow with Hindu Press Ups for ten reps at a medium tempo, Bicycle Crunches for thirty reps at a medium tempo, then Burpees (Non-Jump) variation for eight to ten reps at a high tempo. End with Superman Raises for fifteen reps at a slow tempo. Cool down and finish with some maintenance and/or developmental stretches.

Progressions
Increase the repetitions
Increase the circuits
Decrease the rest period

Bodyweight Circuit 4
To start: Warm-up (see Chapter Three for a detailed description)
Requires: Timer/stopwatch

Exercise	Reps	Tempo	Rest
Squat Kicks	20	High	
Hand to Forearm Press Ups	20	Medium	
Ankle Jumps	20–30	High	
Tuck Jumps	4–6	High	
Elevated Floor Dips	15–20	Medium	
Side Plank Rotator	20	Medium	30–45

Complete two to three circuits.
To finish: Cool down (refer to Chapter Three for a detailed description).

Workout Guide
Start with a warm-up. All the exercises are performed consecutively without rest. The completion of all six exercises constitutes one circuit. Rest thirty to forty-five seconds and repeat for a further one to two circuits. Squat Kicks should be approached at a high tempo for twenty reps (ten kicks per leg), then Elbow-to-Hand Press Ups for fifteen to

twenty reps at a medium tempo, Ankle Jumps for twenty to thirty reps at a high tempo, Tuck Jumps for four to six reps at a high tempo, followed by Elevated Floor Dips for fifteen to twenty reps at a medium tempo. End with Side Plank Rotators for twenty reps (ten per side) at a medium tempo. Cool down and finish with some maintenance and/or developmental stretches.

Progressions
Increase the repetitions
Increase the circuits
Decrease the rest period.

Tabata Workouts (Timed)
Mini-Workout 1: Tabata Single-Exercise High-Intensity Interval
To start: Warm-up (see Chapter Three for a detailed description)
Requires: Timer/stopwatch

Exercise	Sets	Interval (seconds)	Rest (seconds)	Total Time (minutes)
Mountain Climbers	8	20	10	4

To finish: Cool down (refer to Chapter Three for a detailed description).

Workout Guide
Start with a warm-up. Perform as many Mountain Climbers as you can (Level 10 on the RPE chart, page 153) for eight sets of twenty seconds, with ten seconds' rest in between. Cool down and finish with some maintenance and/or developmental stretches.

Progression
Strive at each attempt to work at your maximum intensity

Mini-Workout 2: Tabata Single Exercise High-Intensity Interval
To start: Warm-up (see Chapter Three for a detailed description)
Requires: Timer/stopwatch

Exercise	Sets	Interval (seconds)	Rest (seconds)	Total Time (minutes)
Squats	8	20	10	4

To finish: Cool down (refer to Chapter Three for a detailed description).

Workout Guide
Start with a warm-up. Perform as many Squats as you can (Level 10 on the RPE chart, page 153) for eight sets of twenty seconds, with ten seconds' rest in between. Cool down and finish with some maintenance and/or developmental stretches

Progression
At each attempt, strive to work at your maximum intensity.

Mini-Workout 3: Tabata Single Exercise High-Intensity Interval
To start: Warm-up (see Chapter Three or a detailed description)
Requires: Timer/stopwatch

Exercise	Sets	Interval (seconds)	Rest (seconds)	Total Time (minutes)
Jumping Jacks	8	20	10	4

To finish: Cool down (refer to Chapter Three for a detailed description).

Workout Guide
Start with a warm-up. Perform as many Jumping Jacks as you can (Level 10 on the RPE chart, page 153) for eight sets of twenty seconds, with ten seconds' rest in between. Cool down and finish with some maintenance and/or developmental stretches.

Progression
At each attempt, strive to work at your maximum intensity.

Mini-Workout 4: Tabata Single Exercise High-Intensity Interval
To start: Warm-up (see Chapter Three page xx for a detailed description)
Requires: Timer/stopwatch

Exercise	Sets	Interval (seconds)	Rest (seconds)	Total Time (minutes)
Split Jumps	8	20	10	4

To finish: Cool down (refer to Chapter Three for a detailed description).

Workout Guide
Start with a warm-up. Perform as many Split Jumps (Level 10 on RPE chart) as you can for eight sets of twenty seconds, with ten seconds' rest in between. Cool down and finish with some maintenance and/or developmental stretches.

Progression
At each attempt, strive to work at your maximum intensity.

GPP Workouts (Timed)

Mini-Workout GPP 1

To start: Warm-up (see Chapter Three for a detailed description)
Requires: Timer/stopwatch

Exercise	Sets	Work (seconds)	Rest Between Circuits (seconds)	Total Time (minutes)
Standard Burpees variation	1	30		
Jumping Jacks	1	30		
Squats	1	30		
Alternate Toe Taps	1	30	45–60	
Total				6

Complete two circuits.
To finish: Cool down (refer to Chapter Three for a detailed description).

Workout Guide

Start with a warm-up. Perform Burpees for 30 seconds non-stop at a high intensity (Level 7 on RPE chart). Without resting, move straight onto Jumping Jacks, Squats and Alternate Toe Taps, then rest for 45–60 seconds. The completion of all four exercises constitutes one circuit. Proceed by completing a further circuit. Cool down and finish with some maintenance and/or developmental stretches.

Progressions

Increase the work time
Increase the circuits
Decrease the rest time.

Mini-Workout GPP 2

To start: Warm-up (see Chapter Three for a detailed description)
Requires: Timer/stopwatch

Exercise	Sets	Work (seconds)	Rest Between Circuits (seconds)	Total Time (minutes)
Standard Burpees variation	1	30		
Jumping Jacks	1	30		
Split Jumps	1	30		
Mountain Climbers	1	30	45–60	
Total				6

Complete two circuits.
To finish: Cool down (refer to Chapter Three for a detailed description).

Workout Guide

Start with a warm-up. Perform Burpees for 30 seconds non-stop at a high intensity (Level 7 on RPE chart). Without resting, move straight onto Jumping Jacks, Split Jumps and Mountain Climbers, then rest for forty-five to sixty seconds. The completion of all four exercises constitutes one circuit. Proceed and complete a further circuit. Cool down and finish with some maintenance and/or developmental stretches.

Progressions

Increase the work time
Increase the circuits
Decrease the rest time.

Little Method Workouts (Timed)
Mini-Workout Little Method 1

To start: Warm-up (see Chapter Three for a detailed description)
Requires: Timer/stopwatch

Exercise	Sets	Work Interval (seconds)	Active Rest Interval (seconds)	Total Time (minutes)
Jumping Jacks	8	60	75	17.45

To finish: Cool down (refer to Chapter Three for a detailed description).

Workout Guide
Start with a warm-up. Perform Jumping Jacks for eight sets of sixty seconds at high intensity (Level 7–8 on RPE chart). Active rest for seventy-five seconds between sets with a light jog on the spot (Level 4 on RPE chart). After the final work interval, cool down and finish with some maintenance and/or developmental stretches.

Progressions
Strive to work at a higher intensity during work intervals

Mini-Workout Little Method 2
To start: Warm-up (see Chapter Three for a detailed description)
Requires: Timer/stopwatch

Exercise	Sets	Work Interval (seconds)	Active Rest Interval (seconds)	Total Time (minutes)
High Knees Total	8	60	75	17.45

To finish: Cool down (refer to Chapter Three for a detailed description).

Workout Guide

Start with a warm-up. Perform High Knees for eight sets of sixty seconds at high intensity (Level 7–8 on the RPE chart). Active rest for seventy-five seconds between each set with a light jog on the spot (Level 4–5 on the RPE chart). After the final work interval, cool down and finish with some maintenance and/or developmental stretches.

Progressions

Strive to work at a higher intensity during work intervals

Mini-Workout Little Method 3

To start: Warm-up (see Chapter Three for a detailed description)
Requires: Timer/stopwatch

Exercise	Sets	Work Interval (seconds)	Active Rest Interval (seconds)	Total Time (minutes)
Split Jumps	8	60	75	17.45

To finish: Cool down (refer to Chapter Three for a detailed description).

Workout Guide

Start with a warm-up. Perform Split Jumps for eight sets of sixty seconds at high intensity (Level 7–8 on the RPE chart). Active rest seventy-five seconds between each set with a light jog on the spot (Level 4–5 on the RPE chart). After the final work interval, cool down with some maintenance and/or developmental stretches.

Progressions

Strive to work at a higher intensity during work intervals.

Muscular Endurance Workouts
Mini-Workout: Muscular Endurance
Press Up Ladder 'Chest Challenge'
To start: Warm-up (see Chapter Three for a detailed description)
Requires: Timer/stopwatch

Exercise	Reps	Count	Rest (seconds)
Standard Press Up	1	1	
	2	2	
	3	3	
	4	4	
	5	5	30

Complete two to three circuits.
To finish: re-warm (refer to Chapter Three for a detailed description).

Workout Guide
Start with a warm-up. Perform one Standard Press Up, hold in the 'up' position and count for one. Perform two press ups and count for two in the 'up' position; continue until you reach five reps followed by a five-count. Rest 30 seconds then repeat two to three circuits. Re-warm and finish with some maintenance and/or developmental stretches.

Progressions
Increase the repetitions
Increase the circuits
Decrease the rest

Mini-Workout: Muscular Endurance
Press Up Ladder 'Tricep Challenge'
To start: Warm-up (see Chapter Three for a detailed description)
Requires: Timer/stopwatch

Exercise	Reps	Count	Rest (seconds)
Diamond Press Up	1	1	
	2	2	
	3	3	
	4	4	
	5	5	30

Complete two to three circuits.
To finish: re-warm (refer to Chapter Three for a detailed description).

Workout Guide

Start with a warm-up. Perform one Diamond Press Up, hold in the 'up' position and count for one. Now perform two press ups and count two in the 'up' position. Continue until you reach five reps, followed by a five count. Rest for thirty seconds then repeat two to three circuits. Re-warm and finish with some maintenance and/or developmental stretches.

Progressions

Increase the repetitions
Increase the circuits
Decrease the rest

Mini-Workout: Muscular Endurance

Press Up Ladder 'Upper Chest Challenge'

To start: Warm-up (see Chapter Three for a detailed description)
Requires: Timer/stopwatch

Exercise	Reps	Count	Rest (seconds)
Decline Press Ups	1	1	
	2	2	
	3	3	
	4	4	
	5	5	30

Complete two to three circuits.

To finish: re-warm (refer to Chapter Three for a detailed description).

Workout Guide

Start with a warm-up. Perform one press up, hold in the 'up' position and count one. Now perform two press ups and count two in the 'up' position. Continue until you reach five reps followed by a five count; rest thirty seconds and repeat two to four circuits. Re-warm and finish with some maintenance and/or developmental stretches.

Progressions

Increase the repetitions

Increase the circuits

Decrease the rest

Mini-Workout: Muscular Endurance

'Super Spiderman 30' Circuit

To start: Warm-up (see Chapter Three for a detailed description)

Requires: Timer/stopwatch

Exercise	Reps	Count	Rest (seconds)
Spiderman	2	2	
	4	4	
	6	6	
	8	8	
	10	10	60–90

Complete one to two circuits.

To finish: re-warm (refer to Chapter Three for a detailed description).

Workout Guide

Start with a warm-up. Perform two Spiderman Press Ups, hold in the 'up' position and count for two. Now perform four press ups and count four in the 'up' position; continue until you reach ten reps followed by a ten count. Rest sixty to ninety seconds and strive to repeat a further circuit. Re-warm and finish with some maintenance and/or developmental stretches.

Progressions

Increase the repetitions
Increase the circuits
Decrease the rest

Mini-Workout: Muscular Endurance

Super 'Burpee 55' Circuit

To start: Warm-up (see Chapter Three for a detailed description)
Requires: Timer/stopwatch

Exercise	Reps	Count
Burpee Press Up variation	10	10
	9	9
	8	8
	7	7
	6	6
	5	5
	4	4
	3	3
	2	2
	1	1

Complete one circuit.
To finish: Cool down (refer to Chapter Three for a detailed description).

Workout Guide

Start with a warm-up. Perform ten Burpees then rest for a count of ten. Now perform nine Burpees and rest for a count of nine. Proceed with prescribed reps and corresponding counts until you reach one with a one count. Cool down and finish with some maintenance and/or developmental stretches.

Progressions

Rest for sixty to ninety seconds then attempt another circuit

Core Workouts

Core Workout 1

To start: Warm-up (see Chapter Three for a detailed description)
Requires: Timer/stopwatch

Exercise	Reps	Rest (seconds)
Russian Twists	20	
Seated Row Crunch	10	
Russian Twists	10	
Seated Row Crunch	5	
Reverse Crunches	15	
Side Plank plus Twist	20	
Superman	10	30–45

Repeat circuit three to five times.
To finish: Re-warm (refer to Chapter Three for a detailed description).

Workout Notes

Start with a warm-up. Perform all exercises at a medium tempo without stopping. When performing the Russian Twist and Seated Row Crunch sequence, do not let your feet touch the ground. Take a few seconds' rest and then perform fifteen Reverse Crunches, twenty Side Planks plus Twist (ten per side) and finish with ten Superman. Rest for thirty to forty-five seconds and then repeat the circuit three to five times. Re-warm and finish with some maintenance and/or developmental stretches.

Progressions
Increase the repetitions
Increase the circuits
Decrease the rest

Core Workout 2
To start: Warm-up (see Chapter Three for a detailed description)
Requires: Timer/stopwatch

Exercise	Reps	Rest (seconds)
Bicycle Crunches	20	
V-Ups	10	
Bicycle Crunches	10	
V-Ups	5	
Reverse Crunches	20	
Oblique Crunches Variation 1	20	
Superman	10	30–45

Repeat circuit three to five times.
To finish: Re-warm (refer to Chapter Three for a detailed description).

Workout Notes
Start with a warm-up. Perform all the exercises at a medium tempo without stopping. When performing the Bicycle Crunch and V-Up sequence, do not let your feet touch the ground between exercises. Take a few seconds' rest and then perform twenty Reverse Crunches, twenty Oblique Crunches (Variation 1, ten per side) and finish with ten Superman. Rest for thirty to forty-five seconds and repeat the circuit three to five times. Re-warm and finish with some maintenance and/or developmental stretches.

Progressions
Increase the repetitions
Increase the circuits
Decrease the rest

Core Workout 3
To start: Warm-up (see Chapter Three for a detailed description)
Requires: Timer/stopwatch

Exercise	Reps	Rest (seconds)
Raised Leg Crunch	20	
Cheating V-Ups	10	
Raised Leg Crunch	10	
Cheating V-Ups	5	
Russian Twists	20	
Oblique Seated Row Crunch	20	
Superman	10	30–45

Repeat circuit three to five times.
To finish: Re-warm (refer to Chapter Three for a detailed description).

Workout Notes
Start with a warm-up. Perform all the exercises at a medium tempo without stopping. When performing the Raised Leg Crunch and Cheating V-Up sequence, do not let your feet touch the ground between exercises. Take a few seconds' rest, then perform twenty Russian Twists, twenty Oblique Seated Row Crunches (ten per side) and finish with ten Superman. Rest for thirty to forty-five seconds and repeat the circuit three to five times. Re-warm and finish with some maintenance and/or developmental stretches.

Progressions
Increase the repetitions
Increase the circuits
Decrease the rest

Chapter Seven

LEVEL 3

Important Note: This is the highest level of *5 Minute Fitness* and you must at all costs be conditioned to approach these mini-workouts. Some of the exercises in this chapter represent the most challenging bodyweight exercises available. Also, the overall volume and intensity of the mini-workouts are at a premium.

Level 3 is most suited to the advanced exerciser who may usually attend the gym four to six times per week and for whom fitness plays a major role in their life. Included are GPP, Bodyweight and Tabata workouts, as well as several speed strength mini-workouts. These workouts can be used to supplement your existing programme or maintain and even improve fitness when away or at home. The benefits are consistent throughout and designed to improve your all-round physical fitness.

A number of workouts refer to intensity in the form of Rate of Perceived Exertion (RPE). This method of measuring intensity requires you to self-assess how hard you are working in relation to a numbering system (see page 175). For further information on intensity and how it impacts on your fitness goals, refer to Chapter Two.

You will need a sports timer/stopwatch to complete the timed workouts (the majority of mobile phones have a stopwatch). For Tabata intervals you can download Tabata timers from the Internet (search 'Tabata timer' – there are several to choose from in Google).

Ensure you are wearing appropriate clothing and footwear to exercise in. Do not exercise immediately after eating: allow at least an hour to digest (two hours is ideal and recommended) before. Ensure you have water available.

Where to Exercise

These workouts have been designed to be performed anywhere from your living space to hotel room. Just ensure your exercise area is clear of obstructions and safe to use – check the ceiling height for any jumping that may be involved.

Frequency and Choice of Mini-Workout

Perform one mini-workout per day.

Separate different mini-workouts one day apart and do no more than one Tabata mini-workout per week. You can also add a core mini-workout to any day in addition to your selected workout: perform this immediately afterwards or at a different time during the day.

Example: Five-day week

Monday	Tuesday	Wednesday	Thursday	Friday
Bodyweight Circuit Core Mini-Workout	GPP	Tabata Core Mini-Workout	Bodyweight Circuit	GPP Core Mini-Workout

Borg CR10 Scale

0	Nothing at all
0.5	Extremely weak (just noticeable)
1	Very weak
2	Weak (light)
3	Moderate
4	Somewhat strong
5	Strong (heavy)
6	
7	Very strong
8	
9	
10	Extremely strong
*	Maximal

Feedback on how you feel and how this relates to the scale:

3 Moderate: Easy to perform

4 Somewhat strong: Fairly easy

5 Strong (heavy): Breathing and working a little hard

6 Stronger: Beginning to breathe heavily

7 Very strong: Very challenging, breathing very hard

8 Working and breathing seriously hard

9 Approaching upper limits, working and breathing at near-maximal intensity

10 Extremely strong: Working and breathing at maximal intensity

*Maximal: 100%effort

Important: When using RPE, it is important that you distinguish between the effects of physical fatigue and unsafe signs such as shortness of breath or dizziness, so monitor yourself properly.
Levels of intensity will also be referred to in terms of Tempo Speed, as in the bodyweight circuits (high, medium or low).

Level 3: Mini-Workouts

> **Important:** Please study carefully the information provided at the beginning of this level. If you are new to this kind of rigorous training, take the necessary steps to prepare yourself before starting out. If you have any underlying issues with your health or joint problems, avoid high-intensity and high-impact exercise, which may exacerbate your condition.

Bodyweight Circuits (Reps)

Bodyweight Circuit 1

To start: Warm-up (see Chapter Three for a detailed description)

Requires: Timer/stopwatch

Exercise	Reps	Tempo	Rest (seconds)
Alternate Toe-Taps	20	High	
Tuck Jumps	8–10	High	
Diamond Press Ups	15–20	Medium	
V-Ups	20	Medium	
Jumping Jacks	50	High	
Plyometric Press Ups (Hand Clap)	8–10	High	
Squat Hold	30–45-second count	Static	
Squat Jumps	8–10	High	60–90

Complete two to three circuits.

To finish: Cool down (refer to Chapter Three for a detailed description).

Workout Guide

Start with a warm-up. All the exercises are performed consecutively without rest. The completion of all eight exercises constitutes one circuit. Rest sixty to ninety seconds and repeat for a further one to two circuits.

Alternate Toe-Taps should be approached at a high tempo for twenty reps, then Tuck Jumps for 8–10 reps at a high tempo, Diamond Press Ups for fifteen to twenty reps at a medium tempo, V-Ups for twenty reps at a medium tempo, Jumping Jacks for fifty reps at a high tempo followed by Plyometric Press Ups for eight to ten reps at a high tempo, then into a Squat Hold for forty-five seconds (time or count forty-five). End with Squat Jumps for eight to ten reps at a high tempo. Cool down and finish with some maintenance and/or developmental stretches.

Progressions
Increase the repetitions
Increase the circuits
Decrease the rest period

Bodyweight Circuit 2
To start: Warm-up (see Chapter Three for a detailed description)
Requires: Timer/stopwatch

Exercise	Reps	Tempo	Rest (seconds)
High Knees Plus Skip	60	High	
Prisoner Squats	20	Medium	
Spiderman Press Ups	20	Medium	
Alternate V-Ups	20	Medium	
Lunge Jumps	10	High	
Decline Press Ups	15–20	Medium	
Ankle Jumps	20–30	High	
Plank	30–45-second count	Static	60–90

Complete two to three circuits.
To finish: Cool down (refer to Chapter Three for a detailed description).

Workout Guide
Start with a warm-up. All the exercises are performed consecutively without rest. The completion of all eight exercises constitutes one circuit. Rest sixty to ninety seconds and repeat for a further one to two circuits.

High Knees Plus Skip should be approached at a high tempo for sixty reps, then Prisoner Squats for twenty reps at a medium tempo, Spiderman Press Ups for twenty reps at a medium tempo, Alternate V-Ups for twenty reps at a medium tempo, Lunge Jumps for ten reps at a high tempo, Decline Press Ups for fifteen to twenty reps at a medium tempo, then into Ankle Jumps at a high tempo for twenty to thirty reps. End with a Plank Hold for forty-five seconds (time or count forty-five). Cool down and finish with some maintenance and/or developmental stretches.

Progressions
Increase the repetitions
Increase the circuits
Decrease the rest period

Bodyweight Circuit 3
To start: Warm-up (see Chapter Three for a detailed description)
Requires: Timer/stopwatch

Exercise	Reps	Tempo	Rest (seconds)
Jumping Jacks	50	High	
Burpee Tuck Jump variation	8–10	High	
Dolphin Press Ups	15–20	Medium	
Reverse Crunches	20	Medium	
Wide Squat	15–20	Medium	
Standard Press Up Plus Raised Leg	20	Medium	
Oblique Seated Row Crunches	20	Medium	
Superman	15	Slow	60–90

Complete two to three circuits.
To finish: Cool down (refer to Chapter Three for a detailed description).

Workout Guide

Start with a warm-up. All the exercises are performed consecutively without rest. The completion of all eight exercises constitutes one circuit. Rest sixty to ninety seconds and repeat for a further one to two circuits.

Jumping Jacks should be approached at a high tempo for sixty reps, then Burpee Tuck Jump Variation for eight to ten reps at a high tempo, Dolphin Press Ups for fifteen to twenty reps at a medium tempo, Reverse Crunches for twenty reps at medium tempo, Wide Squat for fifteen to twenty reps at a medium tempo, Standard Press Up Plus Raised Leg for twenty reps (ten reps per leg) at a medium tempo, then into Oblique Seated Row Crunches at a medium tempo for twenty reps. End with Superman for fifteen reps at slow tempo. Cool down and finish with some maintenance and/or developmental stretches.

Progressions

Increase the repetitions
Increase the circuits
Decrease the rest period

Bodyweight Circuit 4

To start: Warm-up (see Chapter Three for a detailed description)
Requires: Timer/stopwatch

Exercise	Reps	Tempo	Rest (seconds)
Mountain Climbers	50	High	
Standard Press Ups	To failure	Medium	
Bulgarian Squat	20	Medium	
Cheating V-Ups	20	Medium	
Burpee Long Jump variation	8–10	High	
Side-to-Side Squats	20	Medium	
Side Plank Plus Twist	20	Medium	
Jumping Jacks	50	High	60–90

Complete two to three circuits.
To finish: Cool down (refer to Chapter Three for a detailed description).

Workout Guide

Start with a warm-up. All the exercises are performed consecutively without rest. The completion of all eight exercises constitutes one circuit. Rest sixty to ninety seconds and then repeat for a further one to two circuits.

Mountain Climbers should be approached at a high tempo for fifty reps, then Standard Press Ups to failure (as many as you can do) at a medium tempo, Bulgarian Squats for twenty reps (ten per leg) at a medium tempo, Cheating V-Ups for twenty reps at a medium tempo, Burpee Long Jump variation for eight to ten reps at a high tempo, Side-to-Side Squats for twenty reps (ten per leg) at a medium tempo, then into Side Plank Plus Twist at a medium tempo for twenty reps (ten per side). End with Jumping Jacks for fifty reps at high tempo. Cool down and finish with some maintenance and/or developmental stretches.

Progressions

Increase the repetitions
Increase the circuits
Decrease the rest period.

Bodyweight Circuit 5

To start: Warm-up (see Chapter Three for a detailed description)
Requires: Timer/stopwatch

Exercise	Reps	Tempo	Rest (seconds)
High Knees	50	High	
Knuckle Press Up	15–20	Medium	
Reverse Lunges	20	Medium	
Burpee Press Up variation	8–10	High	
Floor Dips Plus Extended Leg	20	Medium	
Seated Row Crunches	20	Medium	
Elevated Press Up	15–20	Medium	
Split Jumps	50	High	60–90

Complete two to three circuits.

To finish: Cool down (refer to Chapter Three for a detailed description).

Workout Guide

Start with a warm-up. All the exercises are performed consecutively without rest. The completion of all eight exercises constitutes one circuit. Rest sixty to ninety seconds and repeat for a further one to two circuits.

High Knees should be approached at a high tempo for twenty reps, then Knuckle Press Ups for fifteen to twenty reps at a medium tempo, Reverse Lunges for twenty reps (ten per leg) at a medium tempo, Burpee Press Up variation for eight to ten reps at a high tempo, Floor Dips Plus Extended Leg for twenty reps (ten per leg) at a medium tempo, then into Elevated Press Ups at a medium tempo for fifteen to twenty reps. End with Split Jumps for fifty reps at a high tempo. Cool down and finish with some maintenance and/or developmental stretches.

Progressions

Increase the repetitions

Increase the circuits

Decrease the rest period

Tabata Workouts (Timed)

Mini-Workout 1: Tabata

Multiple Exercise High-Intensity Intervals

To start: Warm-up (see Chapter Three for a detailed description)

Requires: Timer/stopwatch

Exercise	Sets	Interval (seconds)	Rest between sets (seconds)	Rest between exercises (minutes)	Total time (minutes)
Standard Burpees	8	20	10	2	
Jumping Jacks	8	20	10	2	10

To finish: Cool down (refer to Chapter Three for a detailed description)

Workout Guide

Start with a warm-up. Strive to perform as many Burpees as you can (Level 10 on RPE chart) for eight sets of twenty seconds, with ten seconds' rest in between. Rest for two minutes then perform as many Jumping Jacks (Level 10 on RPE chart) as you can for eight sets of twenty seconds, with ten seconds' rest in between. Cool down and finish with some maintenance and/or developmental stretches.

Progressions

Strive to work at your maximum intensity for each attempt
Decrease the two-minute rest between exercises until eventually sixteen sets are performed continuously with no rest between exercises.

Mini-Workout 2: Tabata
Multiple Exercise High-Intensity Intervals

To start: Warm-up (see Chapter Three for a detailed description)
Requires: Timer/stopwatch

Exercise	Sets	Interval (seconds)	Rest between sets (seconds)	Rest between exercises (minutes)	Total time (minutes)
Squats	8	20	10	2	
Mountain Climbers	8	20	10	2	
Total Time					10

To finish: Cool down (refer to Chapter Three for a detailed description).

Workout Guide

Start with a warm-up. Strive to perform as many squats as you can (Level 10 on RPE chart) for eight sets of twenty seconds, with ten seconds' rest in between. Rest for two minutes, then perform as many Jumping Jacks (Level 10 on RPE chart) as you can for eight sets of twenty seconds, with ten seconds' rest in between. Cool down gradually and finish with some maintenance and/or developmental stretches.

Progressions

At each attempt, strive to work at your maximum intensity
Decrease the two-minute rest between exercises until eventually, sixteen
sets are performed continuously with no rest between exercises.

Mini-Workout 3: Tabata
Multiple Exercise High-Intensity Intervals
To start: Warm-up (see Chapter Three for a detailed description)
Requires: Timer/stopwatch

Exercise	Sets	Interval (seconds)	Rest between sets (Seconds)	Rest between exercises (minutes)	Total time (minutes)
Toe Taps	8	20	10	2	
Split Jumps	8	20	10	2	
Total Time					10

To finish: Cool down (refer to Chapter Three for a detailed description).

Workout Guide

Start with a warm-up. Strive to perform as many Toe Taps (Level 10 on
RPE chart) as you can for eight sets of twenty seconds, with ten seconds'
rest in between. Rest for two minutes, then perform as many Split Jumps
(Level 10 on RPE chart) as you can for eight sets of twenty seconds, with
ten seconds' rest in between. Cool down gradually and finish with some
maintenance and/or developmental stretches.

Progressions

At each attempt, strive to work at your maximum intensity
Decrease the two-minute rest between exercises until eventually sixteen
sets are performed continuously with only ten seconds' rest between
each set.

Mini-Workout 4: Tabata
Alternate Multiple Exercise High-Intensity Intervals
To start: Warm-up (see Chapter Three for a detailed description)
Requires: Timer/stopwatch

Exercise	Sets	Interval (seconds)	Rest between sets (seconds)	Rest between circuits (minutes)	Total time (minutes)
Burpees	1	20	10	2	
Standard Squat	1	20	10	2	
Split Jumps	1	20	10	2	
Standard Press Ups	1	20	10	2	
Burpees	1	20	10	2	
Standard Squat	1	20	10	2	
Split Jumps	1	20	10	2	
Standard Press Ups	1	20	10	2	
					10

Complete two circuits.
To finish: Cool down (refer to Chapter Three for a detailed description).

Workout Guide
Start with a warm-up. Strive to perform all the exercises in as many repetitions as possible (Level 10 on RPE chart) consecutively for one set of twenty seconds, followed by ten seconds' rest. Complete eight sets in total, rest completely for two minutes and then repeat the circuit. Cool down gradually and finish with some maintenance and/ or developmental stretches.

Progressions

At each attempt, strive to work at your maximum intensity

Increase circuits

Decrease the two-minute rest between circuits until eventually no rest between circuits is taken

Mini-Workout 5: Tabata

Alternate Multiple Exercise High-Intensity Intervals

To start: Warm-up (see Chapter Three for a detailed description)

Requires: Timer/stopwatch

Exercise	Sets	Interval (seconds)	Rest between sets (seconds)	Rest between circuits (minutes)	Total time (minutes)
Tuck Jumps	1	20	10	2	
Jumping Jacks	1	20	10	2	
Prisoner Squats	1	20	10	2	
Mountain Climbers	1	20	10	2	
Tuck Jumps	1	20	10	2	
Jumping Jacks	1	20	10		
Prisoner Squats	1	20	10	2	
Mountain Climbers	1	20	10	2	
					10

Complete two circuits.

To finish: Cool down (refer to Chapter Three for a detailed description).

Workout Guide

Start with a warm-up. Strive to perform all the exercises in as many repetitions as possible (Level 10 on RPE chart) consecutively for one set of twenty seconds, followed by ten seconds' rest to complete eight sets in total. Rest completely for two minutes and repeat the circuit. Cool down gradually and finish with some maintenance and/or developmental stretches.

Progressions

At each attempt, strive to work at your maximum intensity

Increase circuits

Decrease two-minute rest between circuits until eventually no rest is taken between circuits

GPP Workouts (Timed)

Mini-Workout GPP 1

To start: Warm-up (see Chapter Three for a detailed description)

Requires: Timer/stopwatch

Exercise	Sets	Work (seconds)	Rest Between Circuits (seconds)	Total time (minutes)
Burpees Press Up variation	1	30		
Jumping Jacks	1	30		
High Knees	1	30		
Burpees Press Up variation	1	30		
Jumping Jacks	1	30		
Spiderman Press Ups	1	30	60	
				15

Complete four circuits.

To finish: Cool down (refer to Chapter Three for a detailed description).

Workout Guide

Start with a warm-up. Perform Burpees for 30 seconds non-stop at a high intensity (Level 7 on RPE chart). Without resting, move onto Jumping Jacks, High Knees and then back to Burpees, Jumping Jacks and finish with Spiderman Press Ups. Rest for sixty seconds. The completion of six sets constitutes one circuit: proceed and strive to complete a further three circuits. Cool down and finish with some maintenance and/or developmental stretches.

Progressions

Increase the work time
Increase the circuits
Decrease the rest

Mini-Workout GPP 2

To start: Warm-up (see Chapter Three for a detailed description)
Requires: Timer/stopwatch

Exercise	Sets	Work (seconds)	Rest Between Circuits (seconds)	Total time (minutes)
Burpees Tuck Jump variation	1	30		
Jumping Jacks	1	30		
Split Jumps	1	30		
Burpees Tuck Jump variation	1	30		
Jumping Jacks	1	30		
Diamond Press Ups	1	30	60	
				15

Complete four circuits
To finish: Cool down (refer to Chapter Three for a detailed description).

Workout Guide

Start with a warm-up. Perform Burpees non-stop for thirty seconds at a high intensity (Level 7 on RPE chart). Without resting, move straight onto Jumping Jacks, Split Jumps and back to Burpees followed by Jumping Jacks. Finish with Diamond Press Ups then rest for sixty seconds. The completion of six sets constitutes one circuit. Proceed and strive to complete a further three circuits. Cool down and finish with some maintenance and/or developmental stretches.

Progressions

Increase the work time
Increase the circuits
Decrease the rest

Mini-Workout GPP 3

To start: Warm-up (see Chapter Three for a detailed description)
Requires: Timer/stopwatch

Exercise	Sets	Work (seconds)	Rest Between Circuits (seconds)	Total time (minutes)
Jump Squats	1	30		
Standard Press Ups	1	30		
Prisoner Squats	1	30		
Jumping Jacks	1	30		
Standard Press Ups	1	30		
Prisoner Squats	1	30	60	
				15

Complete four circuits.
To finish: Cool down (refer to Chapter Three for a detailed description).

Workout Guide

Start off with a warm-up. Perform Jump Squats for thirty seconds non-stop at a high intensity (Level 7 on RPE chart). Without resting, move onto Standard Press Ups, Prisoner Squats and Jumping Jacks, then back to Standard Press Ups. Finish with Prisoner Squats once more, then rest for sixty seconds. The completion of six sets constitutes one circuit: proceed and strive to complete a further three circuits. Cool down and finish with some maintenance and/or developmental stretches.

Progressions

Increase the work time
Increase the circuits
Decrease the rest

Mini-Workout GPP 4

To start: Warm-up (see Chapter Three for a detailed description)
Requires: Timer/stopwatch

Exercise	Sets	Work (seconds)	Rest Between Circuits (seconds)	Total time (minutes)
Squat Kicks	1	30		
Jumping Jacks	1	30		
Mountain Climbers	1	30		
Squat Kicks	1	30		
Jumping Jacks	1	30		
T-Press Ups	1	30	60	
				15

Complete four circuits.
To finish: Cool down (refer to Chapter Three for a detailed description).

Workout Guide

Start off with a warm-up. Perform Squat Kicks for thirty seconds non-stop at a high intensity (Level 7 on RPE chart). Without resting, move onto Jumping Jacks, Mountain Climbers and then back to Squat Kicks followed by Jumping Jacks. Finish with T-Press Ups and rest for sixty seconds. The completion of six sets constitutes one circuit: proceed and strive to complete a further three circuits. Cool down and finish with some maintenance and/or developmental stretches.

Progressions

Increase the work time
Increase the circuits
Decrease the rest

Muscular Strength and Power: 'Double Power-Pairs'

To start: Warm-up (see Chapter Three for a detailed description)
Requires: Timer/stopwatch

Exercises	Sets	Reps	Tempo	Rest (seconds)
Pair 1				
(a) Single- Arm Press Ups	4	5 per arm	Medium	
(b) Plyometric Press Ups	4	10	High	60–90
Pair 2				
(c) Isometric Squat	4	Hold for 60 count	Static	
(d) Jump Squats	4	10	High	60–90

To finish: re-warm (refer to Chapter Three for a detailed description).

Workout Guide

Start with a warm-up.

Pair 1: Perform one set of exercise (a) (five reps per arm) immediately followed by one set of exercise (b) for ten reps without stopping. Rest for sixty to ninety seconds and repeat a further three pairs of sets separated by the same rest periods.

Pair 2: Perform one set of exercise (c) for a sixty-count immediately followed by one set of exercise (b) for ten reps without stopping. Rest for sixty to ninety seconds then repeat a further three pairs of sets separated by the same rest periods. Re-warm and finish with some maintenance and/or developmental stretches.

Progressions

Increase the repetitions

Increase the sets

Decrease the rest

Muscular Strength and Power: 'Double Power-Pairs'

To start: Warm-up (see Chapter Three for a detailed description)

Requires: Timer/stopwatch

Exercises	Sets	Reps	Tempo	Rest (seconds)
Pair 1:				
(a) Handstand Press Up	4	5	Medium	
(b) Plyometric Press Up with Chest Slap	4	10	High	60–90
Pair 2:				
(c) Squat Hold	4	Hold for 60 count	Static	
(d) Tuck Jumps	4	10	High	60–90

To finish: re-warm (refer to Chapter Three for a detailed description).

Workout Guide

Start with a warm-up.

Pair 1: Perform one set of exercise (a) for five reps immediately followed by one set of exercise (b) for ten reps without stopping. Rest for sixty to ninety seconds then repeat a further three pairs of sets separated by the same rest periods.

Pair 2: Perform one set of exercise (c) for a sixty-count immediately followed by one set of exercise (b) for ten reps without stopping. Rest for sixty to ninety seconds then repeat a further three pairs of sets separated by the same rest periods. Re-warm and finish with some maintenance and/or developmental stretches.

Progressions

Increase the repetitions
Increase the sets
Decrease the rest

Muscular Strength and Endurance: 'The Special 100 Press Up Challenge'
To start: Warm-up (see Chapter Three for a detailed description)
Requires: Timer/stopwatch

Exercises	Sets	Reps	Tempo	Rest (seconds)
Standard Press Up	1	20	Medium	20
Knuckle Press Up	1	20	Medium	20
Diamond Press Up	1	20	Medium	20
Fingertip Press Up	1	20	Medium	20
Elbow-to-Hand Press Up	1	20	Medium	20

To finish: re-warm (refer to Chapter Three for a detailed description).

Workout Guide

Start with a warm -up. Perform one set of each press-up variation with a twenty-second rest in between. Re-warm and finish with some maintenance and/or developmental stretches.

Progressions

Increase the repetitions
Increase the sets
Decrease the rest

Mini-Workout: Bodyweight Circuit 'Super 300'

To start: Warm-up (see Chapter Three for a detailed description)
Requires: Timer/stopwatch

Exercises	Sets	Reps	Tempo
Standard Press Up	1	25	Medium
Crunches	1	50	Medium
Dolphin Press Up	1	25	Medium
Crunches	1	50	Medium
Decline Press Up	1	25	Medium
Crunches	1	50	Medium
Extended Dip	1	25	Medium
Crunches	1	50	Medium

To finish: re-warm (refer to Chapter Three for a detailed description).

Workout Guide

Start with a warm-up. Perform one set of corresponding reps for each exercise and continue until all the exercises have been completed without rest. Re-warm and finish with some maintenance and/or developmental stretches.

Progressions
Increase the repetitions
Increase the set

Core Workout 1
To start: Warm-up (see Chapter Three for a detailed description)
Requires: Timer/stopwatch

Exercise	Reps	Rest (seconds)
V-Up	20	
Russian Twists	20	
Cheating V-Ups	20	
Reverse Crunch	20	
Side Bridge	20	
Plank Plus Raised Leg	20-second-count hold	30–45

Repeat the circuit three to five times.
To finish: Re-warm (refer to Chapter Three for a detailed description).

Workout Notes
Start with a warm-up. Perform all exercises at a medium tempo without stopping: V-Ups (twenty reps), Russian Twists (twenty reps), Cheating V-Ups (twenty reps), Reverse Crunches (twenty reps), Side Bridges (twenty reps – ten per side) and finish with Plank Plus Raised Leg (twenty seconds or count twenty) per leg raise. Rest for thirty to forty-five seconds then repeat the circuit three to five times. Re-warm and finish with some maintenance and/or developmental stretches.

Progressions
Increase the repetitions
Increase the circuits
Decrease the rest

Core Workout 2

To start: Warm-up (see Chapter Three for a detailed description)
Requires: Timer/stopwatch

Exercise	Reps	Rest (seconds)
Crunch	10 (5 second-count hold	
Russian Twist 20		
Alternate V-Up	20	
Seated Row Crunch	20	
Side Plank Plus Leg Raise	15–20 second-count hold	
Bicycle Crunch	50	30–45

Repeat the circuit three to five times.
To finish: Re-warm (refer to Chapter Three for a detailed description).

Workout Notes

Start with a warm-up. Perform all exercises at a medium tempo without stopping: Crunches (ten reps – hold for five count in the crunch), Russian Twist (twenty reps), Alternate V-Ups (twenty reps), Seated Row Crunch (twenty reps), Side Plank Plus Leg Raise (fifteen to twenty seconds or count fifteen to twenty) per leg raise. Finish with the Bicycle Crunch (fifty reps). Rest for thirty to forty-five seconds, then repeat the circuit three to five times. Re-warm and finish with some maintenance and/or developmental stretches.

Progressions

Increase the repetitions
Increase the circuits
Decrease the rest

Core Workout 3

To start: Warm-up (see Chapter Three for a detailed description)
Requires: Timer/stopwatch

Exercise	Reps	Rest (seconds)
Raised Leg Crunch	25	
Reverse Crunch	20	
Floor Bridge	15	
Oblique Crunch		
Variation II	20	
Side Plank Plus Twist	20	
Plank	45–60-second-count	
Superman	15	30–45

Repeat the circuit three to five times.
To finish: Re-warm (refer to Chapter Three for a detailed description).

Workout Notes

Start with a warm-up. Perform all the exercises at a medium tempo without stopping: Raised Leg Crunch (twenty-five reps), Reverse Crunch (twenty reps), Floor Bridge (fifteen reps), Oblique Crunch Variation II (twenty reps – ten reps per side), Side Plank with Twist (twenty reps – ten reps per side) and Plank Hold for forty-five to sixty (hold for seconds or count). Finish with Superman for fifteen reps. Rest for thirty to forty-five seconds then repeat the circuit three to five times. Re-warm and finish with some maintenance and/or developmental stretches.

Progressions

Increase the repetitions
Increase the circuits
Decrease the rest

A Final Word

Remember, the great thing about these workouts is that they are short in duration and simple to execute; and with all the accompanying benefits, you shouldn't find it too difficult to stay motivated. If they are employed properly, you will feel and see results very quickly.

Try not to contemplate too much – just get on and do the exercises. Soon they will become second nature and part of your daily routine. Excuses such as not having the time, not being able to get to the gym or not being able to find a gym will no longer be valid. Open the book, choose any workout at your level, get your sports gear on, clear a space and get exercising – it couldn't be easier.

Also, remember to listen to your body and if you feel unwell or genuinely too tired, don't force yourself – save your energy for another day as exercise at these times could be detrimental.

It must be acknowledged that, for those who want to make significant gains in specific areas, for example body building, there is a limit as to how far your bodyweight can take you. In addition, if you are specifically training for long-distance activities, mini-workouts would not be sufficient for that goal.

These workouts, however, are a great starting point for those new to fitness and very useful to those who have a good current level of fitness and want to maintain this when away from home. They also make a great addition to existing gym routines.

A BRIEF WORD ON NUTRITION

Here are some basic rules to follow:

- Eat food with nutritional value and cut down on saturated and hydrogenated fats such as butter, hard margarine, fried food, fatty meats, pastry items, cakes, biscuits and chocolate.
- Avoid white foods as best you can (white bread, white pasta etc) as these are processed with no nutritional value.
- Eat good sources of protein (chicken/skinless, fish, pulses etc), carbohydrates (pasta, potato, porridge oats etc) and unsaturated fats (olive oil, flaxseed oil, peanuts, almonds etc).
- Eat little and often if possible (5-6 meals per day) to keep your metabolic rate high and drink a minimum 2 litres of water per day
- Eat 1-2 hours before exercising and eat within 2 hours post-exercise.
- How many calories you eat will depend on what your ultimate goal is: to bulk up, slim down or maintain.

For further information, you can consult these websites:

brianmac.co.uk/nutril.htm

sportsmedicine.about.com/od/sportsnutrition/tp/SimpleSportsNutrition.htm